A WELLNESS GUIDE TO A SPEEDY RECOVERY AND HEALTHY LIVING

Helena A. Prsala, RN and
Helena Prsala, B.Pharm.

Copyright © 2014 by Helena A. Prsala, RN
and Helena Prsala, B.Pharm.

First Edition — October 2014

ISBN

978-1-4602-4115-8 (Hardcover)

978-1-4602-4116-5 (Paperback)

978-1-4602-4117-2 (eBook)

All rights reserved.

No part of this publication may be reproduced in any form, or by any means, electronic or mechanical, including photocopying, recording, or any information browsing, storage, or retrieval system, without permission in writing from the publisher.

Produced by:

FriesenPress

Suite 300 — 852 Fort Street

Victoria, BC, Canada V8W 1H8

www.friesenpress.com

Distributed to the trade by The Ingram Book Company

Table of Contents

Acknowledgments vii
About the authors ix
Introduction 1
    Your Body Talk 2
    Frog Ballad 3
Preparing for hospitalization 7
Healing your body with healthy nutrition 13
    General information 13
    Basic daily requirements 17
    Sample menu 22
Exploring nutrition in greater detail 27
    Important nutrients and their functions 27
    Additional information 36
Exercising your way to greater strength and flexibility 49
    Smile! 53
Attending to mind and spirit 57
    Exercise #1 60
    Exercise #2 60
    Exercise #3 60
    Exercise #4 61
Recuperating at home 65
Promoting good sleeping habits 71
Assisting the patient before, during, and after hospitalization .. 75
    Before admission 76
    During hospitalization 77
    Choosing appropriate gifts 78
    After hospitalization 79
Closing thoughts 81

ADDENDUM

Recipes 85
    Gusto Crepes 86
    Strawberries and cream cheese filling for 4 crepes: 86
    Poultry filling for 4 crepes: 87
    Salmon filling for 4 crepes: 87
    Spinach filling for 4 crepes:. 88
    Mixed vegetables filling for 4 crepes: 88
    Mushroom filling for 4 crepes:. 88
    Fortifying Pulse Soup. 89
    Champion Mushroom Goulash 90
    Two Goodies Soup 91
    Big Apple's Own (Waldorf) Salad. 92
    Highly Vaunted Strudel. 93
    Prune filling:. 94
    Nut filling:. 94
    Spinach filling: 95
    Quick Comfort Bread Pudding 96
    Mini Effort Crumble 97
    Going, Going, Gone Muffins 98
    Invigorating Granola 99
    Pest's Delight Truffles 100
Measurements and conversions 101
Suggested reading 103

Dedicated to all whose knowledge, kindness,
and love inspired us.

Acknowledgments

We extend our profound gratitude to our family for all the loving support, unfailing encouragement, professional input, esthetic insights, and helpful suggestions.

Special appreciation to Jan Prsala Sr., PhD.; Elizabeth Prsala, M.Sc., SLP; Jan Prsala Jr., M.D.; and Janna Mazzarolo, B.Sc. Kinesiology.

Our heartfelt thanks to Trudy Duivenvoorden Mitic, accomplished author and friend, whose invaluable expertise guided our initial efforts.

Thank you to all members of FriesenPress, whose kind assistance made the launch of our book possible.

About the authors

Helena Prsala Sr. is a certified clinical dietitian who received her training in Czechoslovakia and worked there for many years. In Canada, she obtained a nursing diploma from the Halifax Infirmary School of Nursing in Nova Scotia. She worked as a Registered nurse at both the IWK Hospital for Children, and the Halifax Infirmary Hospital. At the latter she served as head nurse of the newly conceptualized Elective Surgery Admission Unit, and later as a volunteer in the Palliative Care Unit. She has also provided nutrition counselling in her own private practice. Helena Sr. experienced first-hand the challenges and duress of surgery and recovery, having undergone several surgeries over the years.

Helena Prsala Jr. graduated with the Bachelor of Pharmacy degree from Dalhousie University in Halifax, Nova Scotia. Her life long interest in wellness originated in childhood having grown up in a family of health and physical education professionals and continued through competitive sports. Helena Jr. is a practicing pharmacist with more than 30 years experience.

Introduction

The primary purpose of this book is to address the needs of a person requiring hospital care, or whose impaired health needs attention. It also benefits his or her family, friends, caregivers, and all who pursue healthy living. The book will guide you through basic practical suggestions to faster recovery and proper health maintenance.

It is extremely important to know what enhances healing. Everyone is unique and complex, comprised of body, mind, and spirit. Taking care of all three components is equally important to your well-being. Your own proactive involvement is essential along with that of the health professionals devoted to your care. Your body is a well- designed, self-healing organism, graciously compensating for various shortcomings that can not be tolerated forever. If you pay attention, you may hear:

Your Body Talk

I am your good buddy,
don't ever doubt,
but sometimes,
when I need your care
I shout,
and make things happen which you may not like.
That's my way to alert you to make them right.
Trust me, my friend,
I always do my best.
Work with me, would you?
We are partners in this quest!

The objective of this book is to assist you in building a solid foundation for the time when your strength and balance need restoring, and to improve your well-being in general. It will help you withstand challenges, be they surgical interventions or conditions requiring medical attention, and also support your future creative realizations.

Stay open-minded and aware of the important role all parts of your being play in establishing and maintaining wellness. In this book there may be segments that do not directly pertain to your situation, or may not be of interest to you presently. Hopefully, you will find the material useful to yourself, or to someone else in the future.

On the same note, the main focus of the nutrition section is on the basic nutritional facts to help your successful recovery. The detailed nutrition section offers additional valuable information to be perused at your leisure.

For a condensed 'refresher course', you may simply review the (soon to be introduced) **PEST**'s promptings, and possibly memorize some of the rhymes. The process of memorizing is always a good workout for the brain.

It is useful to make a list of the ideas that captured your interest so you can return to them later and perhaps cross-reference them with other resources. Your alerted intuition may be signaling the need for a deeper understanding of that particular topic.

If you are reading this book as a patient, acquaint your family, caregivers, and friends with your wellness plan. If you know anyone who would benefit from this book, please share it with him or her, and help apply its principles toward a speedy recovery.

This book reminds you of the universal law of **cause and effect, action and reaction,** and how to use this law to your advantage resulting in better present and future choices.

The following fable summarizes the message of this book .

Frog Ballad

Under a rock wall is a pond
of which the frogs are very fond,
but lately bad news stopped their croaks;
their king is ill and lost all hope.
The realm's esteemed doctor gave advice:
'Majesty, move your precious ass,
jump up high on the rocky wall,
then down to the depth of the waterfall.
For laughs invite your court jester,
be generous, make kind gestures.
Enjoy a sunbath, eat to be well,
trust that all things will soon be swell.'
The king first grumbled, but he jumped,
sun bathed, ate well, and often laughed.
He took his shower in the waterfall,
performed good deeds for the benefit of all.
His health restored, needless to say,
he and his kingdom are happy again.

This simple folk narrative points out that proper care of the entire being — body, mind, and spirit — leads to a successful recovery. Adequate nutrition supplies the components necessary for all body functions. Fresh air provides the much needed oxygen. Sunshine stimulates the production of vitamin D, enhancing immunity. Laughter is great medicine and instills an optimistic frame of mind. Movement promotes circulation resulting in faster healing. Charitable deeds help bring focus on positive aspects of life, nourishing the body, mind, and soul. This overview can serve as a guide while you are recuperating, and beyond.

Throughout the book you will encounter **PEST** (Personal Effort Stimulating Tutor) representing a person's inner voice that he or she often tries to elude rather than seek. The **PEST**'s emphatic prompting can help you along your path to wellness. Also, a time may come to be the **PEST** to others!

Hopefully, you will be pleased to make **PEST**'s acquaintance:

> "Allow me to introduce myself. I am your personal effort stimulating tutor, **PEST** in short, here to encourage you to take self-help action. I am your motivator, health navigator, and goal stimulator. I accept you just the way you are, but I also recognize your full potential. I am the voice of that potential. I support you, and the power within you. I urge you:
>
> Participate,
> be an active member of the health team,
> give it all you can,
> and much faster you will heal.
>
> Please, don't let any other association with the word **pest** tarnish my good intentions. I may be

trying at times, but when I adopt the 'Majesty, move your....' approach it is because I know that it will pay off by expediting your recovery. Are you ready to start?"

We trust that you are ready, and wish you a speedy recovery and healthy living.

Your authors and **PEST**.

Preparing for hospitalization

If possible, become familiar with the self-help ideas in this book before hospital admission.

Your body and mind may be under greater stress at this time and therefore more vulnerable. You need to protect yourself and build your defenses. The following daily intake of supplements, taken with food, can help boost your immune system before, during, and after hospitalization, and maintain good health in the future:

- 1,000 mg vitamin C

- 1,500 mg Omega-3 from marine sources (krill oil, fish oil) or from less potent vegetable sources (chia, hemp, or flax seeds oils)

- up to 2,000 International Units (I.U.) vitamin D3

- 1 multivitamin with minerals

- 1,000–1,500mg calcium with 500–750mg magnesium (Magnesium is needed for efficient utilization of calcium, therefore these two minerals should be taken together in 2:1 ratio. For example: 3 tablets, each containing 333mg calcium and 150mg magnesium, taken daily, for the best results two of the tablets before bedtime).

Before taking any supplements, please confirm with your physician and pharmacist that there are no interactions with your current medications and ask about the best time to take them for optimum effectiveness. Also, be cautious if you have any allergies to foods, medications, or supplements.

Additional preventative measures are listed below.

When exposed to frequent contact with people, take 5mg zinc lozenges (with or without vitamin C and echinacea). Let the lozenge dissolve slowly in your mouth to coat the mucous membranes preventing bacteria and viruses from penetrating the lining of your mouth and throat. Zinc intake should not exceed 60mg per day — including zinc from other sources.

You may choose one from the following supplements: grapefruit seed extract, grape seed extract, oil of oregano, or astragalus. Take the supplement at the manufacturer's recommended dose for at least one week before, during, and for two weeks after hospitalization.

Antibiotics effectively but indiscriminately destroy both bad and good bacteria which may wreak havoc with your digestive system, causing diarrhea, indigestion, and loss of appetite, and may increase the chance of yeast infections. To restore the healthy bacterial flora, take probiotics, such as acidophilus and bifidus (containing at least 80% lactobacillus rhamnosus) three times daily with meals. Alternatively, eat foods rich in active bacterial cultures (though not as concentrated), such as Balkan yogurt, kefir, buttermilk, miso, and sauerkraut, at least two or three times a day in small quantities. Ideally, start one week before, continue during, and for two weeks after finishing the antibiotic therapy.

Beware! Many sneezing, coughing people do not go to doctors; they go to malls, movies, and restaurants. Protect yourself by frequently and consistently washing your hands with soap and water (for at least 15 seconds each time), or at least using hand sanitizer, particularly during flu season, so as not to complicate your recovery or endanger other patients, caregivers, and visitors.

Hydrogen peroxide is an inexpensive, effective disinfectant. Use a mouthful of 3% solution (may be diluted with an equal amount of water) to gargle three times a day, especially in the hospital if possible. Your toothbrush is a potential source of bacteria. Soak it or, at minimum, pour the solution over it after each use. Oral hygiene is very important; the mouth is not only a gateway to wellness, but also illness.

These preventative measures, combined with balanced nutrition and a positive attitude, can stabilize your health and speed up your recovery.

It is helpful to organize yourself before admission. The following is a **list of items to pack:**

- hand sanitizers — to wash your hands when soap and water are not immediately available
- baby wipes — to use after using bed pan, urinal, or commode if soap and water are not within reach
- hydrogen peroxide (3%) — to use as disinfectant
- zinc lozenges — to prevent sore, dry throat
- vitamins and supplements — to provide additional nutritional elements
- lip balm — to prevent dry or chafed lips
- bottled water — to be easily available for your use at any time
- comfortable, front-buttoned night shirt/pajamas — to dress more easily

- bathrobe — to provide warmth and privacy
- front-buttoned or zippered light sweater — to provide additional warmth and comfort
- pair of sturdy slippers — to use for safe walking
- warm socks — to keep your feet warm and cozy
- new toothbrush
- toothpaste
- soap
- facial tissues — to dispose of mucous and sputum secretions
- small pillow — to use for support while coughing, especially if there is an incision on your trunk
- any prescription medications or their comprehensive list, depending on the hospital policy
- ear plugs — to block the noisy hospital activities; let the hospital staff know when you are wearing them!
- entertaining reading or audio material — remember to use earphones

The following is a **list of things to do** before your hospital admission:

- Acquaint yourself, and possibly your family and friends, with the care you will need during your recuperation.
- Prepare several meals and freeze as individual portions.
- Stock up cereal, nuts, raisins, and dried fruit.

- Freeze bread and rolls.

- Practice deep breathing, a simple form of positive visualization, and other suggested exercises.

- Arrange for caregivers by consulting friends, family, and/or local community services.

- Organize any help needed with meals delivery, household chores, pets, mail pick-up, etc.

- Arrange a drive to the hospital.

> **PEST**: "Decide right now that you really want to speed up your recovery and be healthier. Can you envision your better self? Do you like that image? It feels good, doesn't it? Decide to be like that image. Do it now. Be fierce about it. Let it sprout from the very depth of your being. Are you sprouting yet? Affirm that you will do as much as you can for your well-being. Be totally committed. See yourself as new and improved. Good job.
>
> "Picture that you have just ascended one rung on your wellness ladder. This a very important step to creating and maintaining the positive image of your better self. Trust that through discipline and perseverance, you will attain a speedy and successful recovery. I will work diligently with you toward that goal. Count on me to always steady your ladder for your climb.
>
> "Enough prose, let's try this rhyme to sum up:

The Preparation Time

Suck on zinc, and take your 'Cs,'
use the extract of grape seeds.
Oil of oregano is excellent too,
your voyage to health needs this helpful crew.

To keep germs at bay,
gargle merrily away;
salt in water will do well,
so will peroxide of hydrogen.

Wash hands first, then touch your face,
stay away from any close embrace.
Avoid kisses on cheeks and lips,
and acquaint others with these tips.

Nourish your body and the mind,
let positive thoughts lead and guide.
Relax, go the optimistic way,
always expect all to be well."

Healing your body with healthy nutrition

General information

Nutrition influences all body processes. A properly balanced diet can enhance the effect of any therapy, or even be curative of itself. Nutrition as a therapeutic measure was considered very important in ancient times. Egyptian, Jewish, and Greek manuscripts, the original historical sources of medicine, offer valuable insight on the role of nutrition. To quote Hippocrates, the Greek physician of the 5th century BC, "Our food should be our medicine and our medicine should be food," and, "We do not live to eat, we eat to live."

At this point, we would like to mention that our advice on nutrition is primarily for people who do not already follow a specific dietary approach such as nutritarians, vegans, vegetarians, or raw food consumers.

Diversity in your daily intake is important to good nutrition. Plan for a variety of textures, colors, and types of food. This provides a broad spectrum of essential nutrients, and stimulates the appetite that may be poor in time of illness.

All our bodily processes, some more urgently than others, follow a rhythm based approximately on a 24-hour cycle. We therefore need to supply the necessary nutrients regularly. For example, it is no good to skip your vegetables on Tuesday with the promise to gorge on them on Friday. You simply must eat your vegetables (and, by the same token, other required foods) every day.

Eating and drinking at regular intervals ensures proper digestion, absorption, and elimination. All elements necessary for digestion are delivered by blood. Digesting large servings of food is taxing and requires more blood. Large meals, especially high in carbohydrates, cause a sudden increase in blood sugar (glucose) which demands a greater release of the hormone insulin to 'open the doors' for the cells to utilize the sugar. When the job of this doorman is accomplished, the blood sugar level drops just as suddenly, causing one to feel sluggish, tired, and even have a headache.

To minimize unhealthy extremes in blood glucose levels, eat small portions of food at regular intervals (5-6 times daily, including the last snack, no later than one hour before bedtime). It is also important that you limit items high in carbohydrates such as refined flour products, potatoes, rice, and pasta (particularly white), alcohol, and sugar.

Fructose, the sugar found in fruit, fruit juice, and vegetables, does not cause an abrupt increase in blood sugar as does glucose. In small amounts, fructose helps to process glucose properly. However, too much fructose, just as glucose, is converted to fat and can lead to insulin resistance, disabling the body from absorbing glucose normally in the long term. For this reason, eat only small amounts of fruit high in fructose, such as grapes, bananas, mangoes, cherries, apples, pears, pineapples, and kiwis at one time.

Eat slowly and chew well. The first stage of digestion begins in the mouth where chewing increases the production of saliva, moistening the food and releasing the necessary digestive enzymes to start the breakdown of carbohydrates. It is easier for the stomach to handle smaller bites of food allowing better penetration and further digestion by gastric juices. Eating quickly and gulping large chunks of food impairs digestion, leads to air swallowing, and uncomfortable bloating of the stomach. Large amounts of food stay in the digestive tract much longer and could cause abdominal distress. This is especially true when you are ill or recovering, since at this time you may not be up and about with your usual vigor. The lack of mobility and exercise can decrease gastric and intestinal motility.

Focus on adequate fluid intake. Water helps to regulate body temperature, metabolism, osmotic pressure in the cells, and the space between them. Water increases glandular secretions and blood volume, so vitally important particles can be more easily transported where needed. Lack of water can lower blood plasma, thicken the blood, disturb the mineral balance, and threaten normal physiological processes.

Normally, you need at least 2 liters (8 cups) of liquids daily, plus the water contained in solid foods. Before surgery, try to drink an additional 1/2 liter (2 cups) of fluids. If you have a kidney or cardiac condition, always consult your physician before increasing your fluid intake.

During hospitalization, fluid intake is usually monitored and regulated by medical staff, but your understanding and cooperation in this matter is helpful. When you are on your own, continue hydrating regularly. Consider filling a container with 2 liters of water, so you can be assured at the end of the day that you drank your daily requirement. Spring water is preferable to tap water.

The dietitian will arrange a special diet, if needed, while you are in the hospital, and give you instructions to follow at home. If there is no special concern, proper nutrition will be your own responsibility.

Do your best to consume the basic daily requirements outlined later. Consider your individual desires, habits, and tolerance for food, but personal preferences should not be the major determinant of your diet. Nutritional needs have priority. You may occasionally eat something that is not particularly healthy or nutritious just because you enjoy it, but please do not make it habitual.

Counteract temptation with the positive power of your logic, higher mind, and spirit. Don't delay, do it **now**. Concentrate on the present moment, mobilize your powers of positive thinking, and act accordingly. Take it one step at a time, and it will become easier in the next **now**. You have the strength to do it. Picture the rewards accomplishment brings, and apply your self-discipline to realize your vision. In the powerful words of Emile Coue, the famous French pharmacist and psychologist, affirm often, "Every day in every way I am getting better and better," and trust your physical, mental, and spiritual potential.

> **PEST:**
> " 'Are you ready to improve your eating habits?'
> 'It's too late now!'
> 'No, it's never too late.'
> 'O.K., then I have lots of time to think about it.'

Yes, everyone procrastinates sometimes, but now is the time to be strong, renew your promise to achieve a speedy recovery, and follow your good intentions. Be determined to be well, and use your willpower and self-discipline to persevere. Believe me, your efforts will pay off."

Basic daily requirements

If you follow vegetarian, vegan, nutritarian, or raw food diets, then you are familiar with the nutritional requirements of such regimens. As long as your body is doing well on this fare, continue and enjoy.

If you prefer the more traditional dietary approach, you may apply the following nutrition information toward a speedy recovery and beyond.

Proteins, carbohydrates, fats, minerals, vitamins, and fluids are essential for the functioning of our organism. Ideally, the diet is calculated according to a person's age, height, weight, and activity level, but generally the basic nutritional needs are met by the daily consumption of servings indicated below:

- 7 servings of proteins
- 6 servings of vegetables (Carbohydrates I)
- 3-4 servings of fruits (Carbohydrates I)
- 7-9 servings of Carbohydrates II
- 4-5 servings of fats
- 2 liters of fluids

Examples of protein servings — each is approximately equal to 7 grams (g) of protein:

1 oz (28.5 grams) fish, poultry, meat, or venison
6 thin slices oven roasted turkey or chicken
1 large egg
2 tablespoons peanut, almond, or sesame butter
1/4 cup almonds (2 and 1/2 Tbsp)
1/2 cup walnuts
1/2 cup peanuts
1/2 cup cooked legumes (e.g. lentils, beans)

1 cup cooked quinoa
1 cup kefir
1 cup cow's milk
1/3 cup yogurt
1/4 cup dry curds cottage cheese
1 oz gouda, cheddar, mozzarella, or Swiss cheese (with 17% MF: milk fat)
2 oz goat cheese
1/3 can sardines, or wild Pacific sockeye salmon
4 tablespoons flax seed
6 tablespoons Goji berries

Examples of Carbohydrates I servings.

Vegetable servings — each is approximately equal to 5 g of carbohydrates:

1/2 cup cooked asparagus
1/3 cup cooked artichoke
1/2 cup beet greens
1/4 cup sliced raw beets
2/3 cup chopped raw broccoli
1 cup shredded raw cabbage
1 medium carrot
1 cup raw cauliflower
1 cup diced celery
1/2 cup cooked collards
1/2 cup sliced cucumbers
1/2 cup cooked endive
1/2 cup cubed eggplant
1/4 cup raw fiddleheads
1 and 1/2 cups field greens
1/2 cup raw green beans
1/2 cup chopped raw kale
2 cups lettuce in small pieces

2 cups sliced mushrooms
1/4 cup green peas
2/3 cup chopped snow peas
1/2 cup chopped bell peppers
3 tablespoons cooked sweet potato
1 cup sliced radishes
1/2 cup cooked spinach
1 small tomato or 2/3 cup cherry tomatoes
1/2 large zucchini

Fruit servings — each is approximately 18 g of carbohydrates:

1 medium apple
4 medium apricots
1/4 cup dried apricots
2/3 cup canned apricots
1/2 large banana
1 cup blueberries
1 and 1/2 cups blackberries
1 and 1/2 cups cantaloupe
1 cup pitted cherries
3 small pitted dates
1 dried fig
3 tablespoons dried Goji berries
1 medium grapefruit
1 cup grapes
2 kiwis
3/4 cup sliced mango
1 large nectarine
1 large orange
1 cubed papaya
1 large peach
2/3 cup canned peaches
1 small pear
1/2 cup canned pineapple chunks

2 large plums
1/2 pomegranate
4 pitted prunes
2 tablespoons raisins
1 and 1/2 cups raspberries
1 and 3/4 cups watermelon
2/3 cup apple juice
1/2 cup cranberry juice
1 cup grapefruit juice
1/2 cup grape juice
1 cup orange juice

Use the fruit juices and canned products with no additional sugar added.

Examples of Carbohydrates II servings — each is approximately equal to 15 g carbohydrates:

1 thin slice whole grain bread
1/4 bagel, 3 and 1/2" diameter
1/2 English muffin
1 tortilla, 6" in diameter
1/2 Pita, 6" in diameter
2 flat breads (Ryvita, Swedish bread)
1 small roll
1 mini muffin
4 Melba toasts
1/2 cup cooked oats
1/3 cup dry cereal (Raisin Bran)
1/3 cup cooked pasta, or rice
1/2 cup cooked quinoa
1/2 cup mashed potato
1/2 cup cooked pulses (lentils, beans)
3 tablespoons all purpose flour
4 tablespoons coconut, or quinoa flour

3 cups air popped corn
1 tablespoon jam
1 tablespoon honey

Examples of fat servings — each is approximately equal to 5 g of fat:

1 teaspoon butter
1 teaspoon oil
1 teaspoon coconut butter
1/8 cup light cream
1 tablespoon heavy cream
1 tablespoon chopped nuts
1 tablespoon mayonnaise, light
2 slices crisp bacon
1 tablespoon vinaigrette dressing
1/4 avocado
2 and 1/2 tablespoons cream cheese, 15%MF
1/2 tablespoon peanut, almond, sesame butter
1 tablespoon ground flax seeds

For abundant and even energy distribution, consume protein with every carbohydrate intake, including breakfast and snacks.

Check your weight weekly to ensure you do not stray by more than two pounds (1kg) from your normal weight. It is beyond the scope of this book to provide information specifically concerned with weight management.

To summarize: on a daily basis, drink at least 2 liters (8 cups) of fluids, preferably water, eat five to six small meals regularly, and chew slowly and thoroughly. Choose a wide variety of wholesome foods to provide all your basic nutritional requirements, and avoid foods with high carbohydrate and fat content.

Sample menu

The sample menu yields approximately 52 g protein, 63 g fat, 310 g carbohydrates, and 2,000 calories.

Breakfast: 1/4 cup cereal (e.g. oats, wheatlets, millet, quinoa) measured dry, cooked, topped with

1 Tbsp molasses, honey, maple or agave syrup

1 Tbsp freshly ground flax seed

1 cup berries

1 cup of milk (coconut, almond, rice, cow, or goat) may be drunk, or used for cooking or topping cereal

juice, tea, or coffee

Snack: 1/2 apple (peeled and briefly stewed if digesting a raw apple is a problem)

1 Tbsp. nuts

Lunch: asparagus and carrot soup (refer to recipe section)

1 to 2 slices toasted whole grain bread, topped with hummus, sliced tomato, cucumber, lettuce, and 1 to 2 slices of cheese

Waldorf Salad (refer to recipe section)

Snack: 1 whole grain muffin (refer to recipe section)

2/3 cup probiotic plain yogurt

Dinner: 2 to 3 oz (60 to 90 g) cooked fish or poultry

1 cup cooked pasta, rice, rice with beans, quinoa, or mashed potato

2 cups tossed salad

1 cup crisply cooked mixed vegetables

smoothie (1 fruit of your choice, 1/2 Tbsp. flax, hemp, or chia seeds, 1/2 cup light coconut milk, 1/2 tablespoon honey)

Snack: 2 tablespoons homemade granola (refer to recipe section)

1/2 sliced banana

1/2 cup milk of your choice

For additional details on nutrition, please refer to the next chapter, "Exploring nutrition in greater detail."

PEST'S HEALTHY COMBO:

"Veggies, veggies, veggies, fruit, fruit, fruit,
beans, whole grains, nuts and seeds
are all very good.
Naturally raised poultry and wild fish,
eaten sparingly, serve well too.
Feasts of red meat, bad fats, refined flour, and
sugar definitely will not do.
An egg is not a villain and you its prey,
even if you have one every day.
Bring lots of color to your food:
red, orange, purple, green, and blue.
Don't forget eight cups of fluids or more,
with healthy foods aim for wellness, and score!
Nutritarians, vegans, vegetarians, raw food fans,
follow the rules your diet recommends.
With a wide variety of balanced foods,
march to your drum on familiar routes
and since you found the way to be satisfied,
keep going and have a happy ride.

"Please use this poem as an inspiration, and focus daily on your nutritional goals. Hold nature's gift of food in reverence, since it is one of the major tools for restoring and maintaining health.

"You need plenty of liquids to hydrate your body. To answer your trick question, yes, alcohol is a liquid, but while water cleanses, hydrates, and makes every cell in your body quiver with pleasure, this cannot be said about alcoholic beverages. You may experience an initial bodily quivering, but no cleansing and hydrating.

Alcohol is actually a diuretic, and its excessive consumption can cause dehydration. One glass of wine or beer daily is acceptable as long as it does not interfere with your medical condition or medications.

Remember, the focus is on your nutritional needs, so you primarily need water. Herbal teas and juices (preferably unsweetened and/ or diluted with water) may also be consumed to seal the purifying deal.

On that note, I bid you happy eating and drinking.

"Here is a dose of humor:

As an experiment, the teacher places a worm in a glass of water. The worm seems to be quite happy, writhing about, doing somersaults, enjoying his environment. The

teacher now places another worm in a glass of whiskey. It is very obvious that the worm is not a happy camper, and shortly sinks to the bottom, dead.

'What lesson did we learn from this experiment?' asks the teacher.

'I know, I know!' one pupil exclaims. 'If you drink whiskey, then you won't get worms!'

"Ready for another one?

'Do you drink to excess?'

'I drink to everything.'

(Water, of course, what else?)

"How are you doing so far climbing your wellness ladder? Be objective, not overly critical or too generous. Is there any area where you need to push harder, or conversely, take it easy? Evaluate your progress from time to time. This will help to direct your path, focus your effort, and encourage your perseverance."

Exploring nutrition in greater detail

Important nutrients and their functions

Proteins are composed of amino acids and perform three main functions. They serve as the material for growth and repair of cells, partial composition of hormones and enzymes, and storage of energy.

Complete proteins contain all amino acids and are found in foods such as milk, milk products, eggs, fish, meats, and poultry. Incomplete proteins lack some amino acids and are found in plants, of which nuts, soy, and legumes are the best sources. Vegetables, fruits, breads, and cereals also provide a small amount of proteins.

Carbohydrates consist of simple and complex sugars, and starches. They provide energy for the activities of all body cells, and heat production.

The main sources of carbohydrates are grains (barley, quinoa, oats, rice, rye, wheat), sugars, honey, syrups, molasses, vegetables, and fruits. Glycogen, or so-called animal starch, is found in liver and seafood. Milk also contains some carbohydrates in the form of the sugar lactose.

Fats are composed of fatty acids, the main source of energy in the body. Fats produce two and a half-times more energy than proteins and carbohydrates. The deposits of fat under the skin decrease the dissipation of body heat and help maintain even body temperature. Fatty acids are necessary for the synthesis of cells and help the absorption of vitamin A, D, E, and K, as well as some minerals.

Saturated fats come from animal sources (pork, beef, venison) and their byproducts (butter, lard, suet). They are solid at room temperature. Fat found in poultry is considered intermediate in the content of saturated fatty acids.

Tropical oils, such as coconut and palm kernel oils, are also classed as saturated fats but differ in their chemistry from animal fat. They affect the immune system positively, and lower the risk of coronary diseases. The body best utilizes tropical oils and monounsaturated fats.

Monosaturated fats originate from plants (nut, seeds, and olive oils, avocados) and exist in liquid or semi-solid form. They have a common feature with saturated fats: they do not oxidize easily. They are known to raise HDL (high density lipids, the good fats), and lower LDL (low density lipids, the bad fats), protecting the circulatory system.

Polyunsaturated fats are in soy, corn, safflower, canola, and cottonseed oils. They are the most unstable form of fats, oxidize easily, readily become rancid, and thus create free radicals (agents causing tissue damage at cellular level).

Minerals perform a variety of vital metabolic functions. The most important minerals are: calcium, chromium, copper, iodine, magnesium, phosphorus, potassium, sodium, sulfur, and zinc. When calcium, phosphorus, iron, and iodine are supplied from food sources, the other minerals are also likely to be present.

The following recommended daily intake values are quoted for adults.

C a l c i u m is essential to the growth, development and maintenance of bones and teeth. It helps to regulate heartbeat, blood pressure, clotting of blood, responsiveness of neuro-muscular systems, enzyme activation, and cell wall permeability. Calcium is best absorbed and utilized in the presence of carbohydrates, proteins, vitamin D, magnesium, and zinc. The recommended daily intake ranges between 1,000mg to 1,500mg and, as mentioned previously, the ratio between calcium and magnesium should ideally be 2:1. The main sources of calcium are milk and milk products. Green leafy vegetables, broccoli, nuts, and grains also provide substantial amount of calcium.

C h r o m i u m assists in the metabolism and storage of proteins, carbohydrates, and fats. It enhances the action of insulin. Vitamins C and B1 increase absorption of chromium. The minimum daily recommended value is 30mcg. Food sources of chromium are vegetables (namely broccoli), fruits, and whole grain products.

C o p p e r helps the body utilize iron, and form blood cells and connective tissues. The usual recommended daily intake is about 1mg per day. Food sources of copper are liver, oysters, lobster, calamari, seeds (sunflower, flax, sesame, pumpkin, squash), tahini (sesame butter), dark chocolate and cocoa, nuts, sun dried tomatoes, and dried herbs.

I o d i n e is important for the function of the thyroid gland. Thyroid gland hormones regulate metabolism, energy, temperature, and reproduction. The average daily recommended intake is about 150mcg. Dietary sources of iodine are iodized salt, seaweed (kelp), fish, and potato with the skin left on.

I r o n is needed for red blood cell production, muscle formation, transportation of oxygen, and energy. The recommended intake values vary from 8 to 18mg per day. The followers of vegetarian and vegan regimens should have at least 40mg of iron daily. Food sources of iron are red meat, poultry, liver, clams, mussels, oysters, shrimp, dark green leafy vegetables, kale, broccoli, yellow beans, spirulina, tofu, pistachios, sesame seeds, fortified breads, and cereals.

M a g n e s i u m is very important for maintaining regular heartbeat and normal functioning of muscles, nerves, bones, and the immune system. The minimum daily recommended intake is about 400mg. Good food sources are bran (oat, rice, wheat), nuts (particularly Brazil nuts, cashews, walnuts, and almonds), seeds, oatmeal, dates, raisins, molasses, soybeans, peanut butter, low fat yogurt, chocolate, lentils, bananas, and brown rice.

Phosphorus plays a complementary role to calcium in bone and tooth formation. This mineral is also needed in the metabolism of carbohydrates and fats and is essential in a variety of chemical reactions in the body. The recommended daily intake is about 800mg per day. Good sources are milk and milk products, eggs, lean meats, legumes, grains, and nuts. If calcium intake is adequate, then usually so is the intake of phosphorus.

Potassium is a crucial element associated with cell metabolism, fluid and acid-base balance. It has a significant effect on muscle activity, especially the heart, by transmitting electro-chemical impulses. Potassium is also necessary for protein formation. The recommended daily intake is not firmly established but 4,500mg is suggested presently. Patients taking diuretics or heart medications should be aware whether these drugs are potassium sparing or depleting, so their potassium level remains stable.

Almonds, dried fruits, nuts, avocado, brussels sprouts, yams, sardines, halibut, molasses, bitter chocolate, chard, garden cress, peanut butter, potatoes, and cereals are good sources of potassium.

Sodium is indispensable for regulating the water balance, maintaining all cells in a healthy state, transporting nutrients, and transmitting nerve impulses. The requirement for sodium is not firmly established. There are many factors involved in determining individual needs but 1,000mg to 1,500mg per day (2/3 of a teaspoon) is the agreed upon recommended range. The most common sources of sodium are table salt, baking soda, condiments, seasonings, monosodium glutamate (MSG), smoked meats, pickled foods, fish, poultry, dairy products, and eggs.

Zinc is needed for the production of proteins, enzymes, hormones, and the proper function of the reproductive system.

It assists in healing, keeping the immune system strong. It also maintains normal sense of taste and smell. The recommended daily intake is 10-15mg per day (the lower value for females). The dietary sources of zinc are oysters, crab, veal liver, beef, lamb, wheat germ, peanuts, pumpkin and squash seeds, cocoa, and dark chocolate.

Vitamins are protective factors important for the optimal function of our organism. Vitamins fulfill the task of biological catalysts and as such help to regulate metabolic processes. There are two groups of vitamins: fat-soluble (A, D, E, K) and water-soluble (B complex, vitamin C).

V i t a m i n A helps to maintain good vision, healthy skin, proper condition of mucus membranes (the lining of air passages and gastrointestinal and genitourinary tracts), fight infection, build bones, and support growth. Recommended daily intake is 5,000 to 10,000 I.U. The precursor of vitamin A is beta-carotene; the body converts beta-carotene into vitamin A. Food sources are dark green, red, orange, and yellow vegetables, yellow fruit, fish oils, whole milk and dairy products, butter, liver, and egg yolk.

Cholesterol lowering medications (cholestyramine, colestipol), or mineral oil (taken on regular basis for constipation) can reduce blood levels of dietary beta-carotene.

Deficiency of vitamin A manifests in a weakened immune system, skin problems (scaly patches), hair loss, and, in severe cases, night blindness or loss of vision.

V i t a m i n D (particularly its most active form, D3), enhances absorption and utilization of calcium and phosphorus needed for bone and tooth formation and maintenance. It prevents rickets, a condition when bones become weak resulting in arms and legs bowing. Vitamin D also helps to build immunity. The recommended daily intake is 1,000 I.U and even higher doses may be used in severe deficiencies, or for persons over 70 years old.

Dietary sources are mackerel, salmon, tuna, fish oils, in smaller amounts milk, dairy products, egg yolk, butter, and liver. Another source of vitamin D is the sun; the ultraviolet rays trigger the chemical process in the skin to produce this vitamin. To a lesser extent, vitamin D is also created with the help of bacteria in the intestines.

Deficiency of vitamin D could cause discomfort in bones, osteoporosis, muscle weakness, insomnia, diarrhea, and a weakened immune system.

V i t a m i n E is important for the integrity of cell membranes, red blood cell formation, glandular function, vitamin K utilization, its anti-inflammatory and antioxidant properties, and the health of the immune system. The recommended daily intake is approximately 200 I.U. to 400 I.U. If you are taking blood thinners, consult your physician before starting or discontinuing vitamin E supplement, since it may affect the efficacy of these medications. For best effectiveness, a vitamin E supplement should contain all the tocopherols — alpha, beta, gamma, and delta (check the label). Vitamin E is found in wheat germ, nuts, seeds (particularly sunflower seeds), green leafy vegetables, legumes, soy beans, fortified cereal, egg yolk, kiwi, and mango.

People who have a problem absorbing fats properly (in Crohn's disease, cystic fibrosis, or inability to secrete bile) may show vitamin E deficiency symptoms such as muscle weakness, balance problems, nerve problems, and impaired vision. They may require water soluble vitamin E.

V i t a m i n K is essential for normal blood clotting. It has the opposite function from blood thinners, so people on these medications should not consume large amounts of foods rich in vitamin K, and vitamin K supplements should also be avoided. The recommended daily intake is approximately 100mcg a day. Food sources are kale, collards, spinach, turnip, beet and mustard greens, brussels sprouts, broccoli, romaine lettuce, parsley, asparagus, cabbage, and sauerkraut.

Deficiency of this vitamin is relatively rare, but can cause problems in blood clotting manifesting as nosebleeds, bleeding gums, heavy menstrual bleeding, and blood in the urine and stool.

Vitamin B complex (B1, B2, B3, B5, B6, B7, B9, B12). B vitamins work in unison; therefore if supplementing, it is important to take them all together as the B complex. Even if a higher dose of a specific B vitamin is needed, the basic amount of the B complex should also be taken. It is best to choose an equalized formula where all the B vitamins have the same dosage. The minimum recommended daily dose is 15mg with the exception of folic acid, biotin, and B12.

B vitamins are important in enhancing the immune system, keeping the nervous system, skin, and muscles in healthy condition, promoting cell function, and supporting normal intestinal activity. A good source of all B vitamins is brewer's yeast.

Take B vitamins with meals or after meals, not on an empty stomach as this could cause gastro-esophageal reflux or nausea. B vitamins will turn urine bright yellow.

Vitamin B1, thiamine, is needed for proper utilization of carbohydrates and proteins. It strengthens the heart, activates the appetite, promotes healthy nerve cells formation, and normal activity of neurotransmitters for muscles and nerves. Dietary sources are organ meats, brewer's yeast, whole grains and enriched cereals, eggs, wheat germ, nuts, legumes, and berries.

Vitamin B1 deficiency presents as tiredness, indigestion, loss of appetite, and muscle discomfort. Alcoholism is the leading cause of B1 deficiency.

Vitamin B2, riboflavin, is engaged in the metabolism of proteins, carbohydrates, and fats, healthy function of heart, red blood cell production, healthy skin maintenance, and prevention of cataract onset and light sensitivity of the eyes. It also helps create favorable conditions for the utilization of the other B vitamins. Good sources of vitamin B2 are yeast, organ meats, venison and other red meat, eggs, milk, leafy vegetables, mushrooms, and enriched cereals.

Vitamin B2 deficiency manifests as sores on lips, tongue and mouth, and as cracks at the corner of the mouth.

Vitamin B3, niacin (also known as nicotinic acid, vitamin P, PP, or anti-pellagra factor), is necessary for healthy skin, and prevention of insomnia and atherosclerosis (the condition where plaque adheres to the arteries). It also helps the body derive energy from proteins, carbohydrates, and fats. Sources of vitamin B3 are chicken, liver, salmon, halibut, yeast, nuts, legumes, whole grains, and enriched cereals.

Severe deficiency of vitamin B3 can cause pellagra, a condition affecting the digestive and nervous systems, and the skin. Alcoholism can also lead to pellagra.

Vitamin B5, pantothenic acid, plays an important role in the metabolism of proteins, carbohydrates, and fats, energy production, and hormone synthesis. It maintains a healthy central nervous system, relieves heartburn, minimizes allergies, and prevents fatigue. Organ meats, chicken, yogurt, eggs, corn, and yeast are the richest sources of this vitamin.

Deficiency is rare because vitamin B5 is abundant in both the animal and plant kingdoms. If it does occur, it manifests as muscle cramps, numbness in the limbs, and a burning sensation on the tongue.

Vitamin B6, pyridoxine, is needed for proper function of the body in general. It maintains a healthy central nervous system, liver, skin, eyes, mouth, hair, immune system, and hormonal balance. Vitamin B6 protects arterial linings and the heart. It helps to form red blood cells, convert food to energy, and prevent convulsive seizures. Good dietary sources are bran (wheat and rice), whole grains, raw pistachios, raw garlic, lean pork, liver, fish, sesame and sunflower seeds, bananas, hazelnuts, molasses, Sorghum syrup, spinach, and potatoes with skin.

Deficiency of this vitamin can result in skin problems, anemia, depression, tiredness, and possibly kidney stones.

Vitamin B7, biotin (also called vitamin H), is required for the synthesis of fatty acids, the release of energy from carbohydrates, the utilization of vitamin B12, and healthy maintenance of nails and hair.

Recommended daily intake is approximately 30mcg. Food sources of biotin are egg yolk (raw egg white impairs biotin absorption), broccoli, cabbage, cauliflower, avocado, green leafy vegetables (best eaten raw as cooking depletes biotin), brewer's yeast, beef, chicken, fish, nuts, grains, liver, and kidney.

Deficiency of B7 is rare, but can happen if the intestinal bacteria that create this vitamin are destroyed, for instance, by the frequent use of antibiotics. The symptoms are susceptibility to infections, muscle strain, fatigue, skin problems, depression, and hair loss.

Vitamin B9, folic acid (folate, vitamin M or B-c), is essential for fetal development, red blood cell and amino acid formation, cell health, normal function of the gastrointestinal tract, protein metabolism, and the prevention and treatment of anemia, sprue, heart disease, and possibly even cancer.

The minimum daily requirement is 400mcg, although women planning pregnancy or pregnant need to take minimum 1mg daily. Alcoholics and patients on methotrexate require minimum 5mg daily. Dietary sources are asparagus, green leafy vegetables, beets, legumes, nuts, citrus fruit, bananas, brewer's yeast, organ meats, poultry, pork, shellfish, salmon, tuna, wheat bran, barley, fortified cereals, and milk.

Deficiency of folic acid can lead to anemia, fatigue, infertility, birth defects, insomnia, depression, gastrointestinal problems, palpitations, and confusion.

Vitamin B12, cobalamin or cyanocobalamin, is extremely important in red blood cell production, their healthy shape and proper function. It plays a crucial role in the treatment of anemias (mainly pernicious). It maintains a healthy nervous system. Minimum recommended daily intake is 2.4mcg. If supplementation is needed, the dose may vary from 100 to 1200mcg depending on the medical condition. Vitamin B12 is poorly absorbed in Crohn's or Celiac disease, or if part of the stomach is removed. Diabetes medication metformin and alcoholism deplete vitamin B12. Food sources are liver, beef, lamb, nutritional yeast, clams, oysters, mussels, crab, lobster, fish, eggs, milk, cheese, and leafy vegetables.

Deficiency of B12 causes anemias, fatigue, depression, confusion, memory loss, gastrointestinal problems, loss of appetite, dizziness, sore tongue and mouth, numbness and tingling in the hands.

Inositol and choline are usually grouped with B vitamins but are not actually categorized as such.

Inositol helps to establish healthy cell membranes, maintain proper nerve impulses, stabilize mood swings, assist in the breakdown of fats, increase the HDL levels, and improve insulin sensitivity. Minimum daily allowance is approximately 1.5mg. Higher intake could cause gastrointestinal problems. Food sources are wheat bran, nuts, seeds, fruits, brown rice, and corn.

Choline maintains healthy cell membranes, protects liver from fat accumulation, lowers cholesterol, prevents birth defects, and possibly memory loss with aging, and may help control asthma. The suggested daily intake is 500mg. Intake of 3gm or more produces side effects such as low blood pressure, diarrhea, and unpleasant body odor. The dietary sources are liver, eggs, soybeans, beef, butter, peanuts, seeds, wheat germ, cauliflower, spinach, grains, legumes, and fish.

Additional information

Our body pH (power of hydrogen) should be slightly alkaline, 6.2 to 7.4 (the lower the pH, less than 7, the more acidic; the higher the pH, the more alkaline). Excessive acidity in the body provides a favorable environment for many disease states such as arthritis, heart and digestive problems, osteoporosis, and cancer. Our diet should contain 75 to 80% alkaline-forming foods and 20 to 25% acid-forming foods.

A highly alkaline environment is produced by honeydew, watermelon, nectarine, raisins, raspberries, fresh black cherries, pumpkin seeds, almonds with skin, plain almond butter, all sprouts, baking soda, sea salt, dairy-free probiotic cultures, soy lecithin granules, black olives, miso, and ginkgo biloba.

A medium alkaline environment is produced by cauliflower, sweet potato, cabbage, celery, carrots, parsnip, endive, asparagus, bell pepper, lemon, lime, pink grapefruit, apple, avocado, pear, peach, mango, chestnuts, Brazil and macadamia nuts, aloe vera juice, flax seed, extra virgin olive oil, black current oil, green, ginger, camomile, and rooibos teas, regular, ozonated or ionized water, pure omega-3 fish oil, dairy probiotic cultures, whey protein, apple cider vinegar, blackstrap molasses (without sulfur), cinnamon, dill, mint, turmeric, ginger, oregano, basil, ginseng, and peppermint.

A low alkaline environment is produced by brussels sprouts, tomatoes and tomato juices, beets, mushrooms, potatoes with skin, squash, pumpkin, fresh peas, lettuce, tempeh, blueberries, blackberries, strawberries, grapes, papaya, apricots, fresh pineapple, whole oats, wild rice, quinoa, spelt, millet, hemp seeds and oil, flaxseed, sesame seeds and oil, sunflower seeds and oil, fresh coconut and oil, goat cheese (soft), fresh goat milk, cod liver oil, brown rice syrup, raw honey, pure maple syrup, stevia, dry red wine, draft beer or dark stout, unsweetened almond milk, organic black coffee, distilled water, curry, mustard powder, most herbs, tamari, maca, astragalus, echinacca, and milk thistle.

Highly acid forming foods are salted, sweetened peanut butter, trans fatty acids, cakes, pastries, cookies, processed soybeans, soy sauce, processed cheese, hard cheese, egg yolk, pistachios, barley, alcoholic drinks, soft drinks, beef, lobster, cranberries, sulfured dried fruit, white vinegar, MSG, brewer's and nutritional yeast, and artificial sweeteners.

Medium acid forming foods are salted, unsweetened peanut butter, pecans, walnuts, cashews, rolled oats and oat bran, rye, white pasta, white bread, white rice, rice protein powder, chicken, lamb, pork, veal, soft cheese, soy cheese, whole eggs, prunes, sweetened fruit juice, jams, preserves, canned fruit, corn syrup, fructose, sugar, coffee with milk and sugar, ketchup, mayonnaise, nutmeg, vanilla, and balsamic vinegar.

Low acid producing foods are peanuts with skin, organic peanut butter (unsalted, unsweetened), pine nuts, dried beans, lentils, green peas, split peas, chick peas, soy protein powder, corn, firm tofu, tahini, cocoa, carob, regular salt, unsweetened soy and rice milk, black tea, black and decaf coffee, dried fruit, natural figs, dates, banana, unsweetened jams and preserves, natural fruit juices, unsweetened canned fruit, popcorn, canola oil, grape seed oil, green soybeans, brown and basmati rice, wheat, buckwheat, whole wheat and corn pasta, whole grain bread, kasha, amaranth, fish, seafood, turkey, duck, venison, cow's milk, yogurt, butter, cream, buttermilk, egg white, rice vinegar, and commercial honey.

Extensive handling of fruits and vegetables, long transportation time from harvest to market, and long cooking time diminish their quality and nutritional value. The use of pesticides is obviously not good either. Therefore fresh, locally grown, organic fruits and vegetables are the best choices for you, followed by non-organic fresh, organic frozen, non-organic frozen, and finally organic and non-organic canned produce.

Before eating or cooking, wash all fruits and vegetables thoroughly under running water and dry them. To reduce the content of pesticides, soak non-organic produce in a solution of organic raw apple cider vinegar (two tablespoons) and water (1 liter, or 4 cups) for ten minutes, then rinse under running water. Grape or grapefruit seed extract or Fruit and Veggies soak (a vegan product) solutions are alternate options for the removal of contaminants. Follow the label instructions. Some B and C vitamins may be lost during this process, but you can obtain them from other sources. That's another reason why variety is important in your diet.

High content of pesticides (estimated presently) has been found mainly in celery, kale, collards, potatoes, peppers, spinach, lettuce, apples, strawberries, grapes, nectarines, peaches, plums, and cherries.

The least contamination (estimated presently) has been found in onion, corn, asparagus, sweet pea, sweet potato, mushrooms, eggplant, cabbage, broccoli, tomatoes, pineapple, avocado, mango, watermelon, grapefruit, papaya, and kiwi.

Salt and sugar are often added to canned goods, so rinse them well under running water. Check the labels and choose the canned fruit preserved in its own juice or at least in light syrup. Bisphenol A (BPA) prevents corrosion of metal and preserves food, but it is a chemical additive. Therefore, whenever possible, choose canned foods that are labeled 'BPA free.'

Have some green, yellow, orange, and red vegetables every day. Recent research indicates that many vegetables (such as root vegetables, cabbage, cauliflower, broccoli, tomatoes, mushrooms, spinach, and zucchini) release their nutrients better when lightly cooked rather than raw.

Steam or stirfry vegetables briefly to eat them when they're crisp, not mushy. Don't discard the cooking water; use it as stock. Cook frozen produce quickly without thawing, as it was probably already blanched before packaging. The nutritional value of frozen products diminishes over time, but up to six months is acceptable.

Legumes, also known as pulses (beans, lentils, peas), are very valuable members of the food family due to their protein and fiber content. Have them at least a couple times a week. Eat other fiber-rich foods like whole grain products, vegetables, fruits, nuts, and seeds daily.

If you choose to eat red meat, doing so once every ten days is acceptable. Poultry and fish are easier to digest, but limit even their consumption to twice a week. If possible, buy naturally raised poultry, beef, pork, or bison with no hormones or antibiotics added. Do not indulge in smoked products since they may contain carcinogens (cancer-causing or -aggravating substances).

One of the tasks of the liver is to detoxify the body from harmful substances. It is wise not to eat the liver of animals and birds, particularly if they are fed antibiotics, hormones, or other unnatural additives since they could contaminate your system and cause your liver to work harder.

Wash (or even soak for five minutes) meats, poultry, and fish in the above-mentioned apple cider vinegar solution, and then rinse under cold, running water before cooking to remove possible pollutants and unwanted microbes.

Read labels and avoid foods containing hydrogenated or partially hydrogenated fats (including trans fats). Beware of cookies, crackers, and deserts that contain these fats. Cut back on saturated fats from animal sources, but you may enjoy a small amount of butter, preferably from grass-fed cows, i.e. Organic Valley pasture butter, Kerrygold pure Irish butter, Anchor butter, Kalona Organic butter...

Salmon (fresh wild Pacific is the best), sardines, mackerel, halibut, herring, and anchovies are sources of healthy fats. Other sources are coconut butter and oil, cold pressed oils (walnut, flax seed, sesame seed, extra virgin olive, palm, and macadamia nut oils), nuts, seeds, nut butters, and avocados. Gout sufferers should avoid anchovies, sardines, pickled herring, and nuts to prevent flare-ups.

Omega-3 fatty acids are beneficial in the prevention and treatment of cardiovascular disease and immune system disorders. These fatty acids are abundant in the above mentioned seafood, walnuts, macadamia nuts, flax, chia, psyllium, and hemp seeds, omega-3 fortified eggs, spinach, broccoli, cauliflower, winter squash, and beans. To be fully absorbed and utilized, flax and psyllium seeds should be ground and consumed fresh, but may be refrigerated for several days. Omega-3 fatty acids loose their value when exposed to heat. Whole flax and psyllium seeds in baked goods pass through the digestive system without being properly broken down and absorbed, in which case they are only useful as fiber.

Omega-3s can be taken as supplements, best sourced from wild salmon, anchovy, sardines, mackerel, or krill oil. Caution must be used with these supplements as they thin the blood, increasing bruising and bleeding. This is especially a concern for anyone already taking anticoagulants such as warfarin, clopidogrel, or acetylsalicylic acid (ASA). Do not use fish or krill oil before surgery. If you are a diabetic, blood sugar levels may be affected also, so test carefully when using flax seed and omega-3 supplements. Breast, uterine, and prostate cancer patients are advised to avoid flax seed due to its estrogen-like properties.

Every oil has a different smoke point that needs to be taken in consideration when cooking. As soon as smoke appears, carcinogens are released in the air, and free radicals are released from the oil. Both are dangerous to our health. The higher the smoke point, the safer is the oil. Cold-pressed oils are always the best (labeled also as 'unrefined,' or 'expeller-pressed').

Extra virgin olive oil and flax seed oil, due to their low smoke points, are preferable for salad dressings, marinades, dips, and light sauteing. Flax seed oil is not shelf stable; check it often for freshness. Walnut and grape seed oils have a medium to high smoke point good for sauteing and baking. Peanut and sesame oils and pure non-hydrogenated lard have a high smoke point, so can be used for cooking, even for frying, but remember, frying is generally discouraged. Use all oils and animal fats in small amounts only. Avoid safflower, corn, sunflower, cottonseed, soy, and canola oils; they readily create free radicals. Coconut oil is, according to contemporary research, the best for all cooking needs.

Omega-6 fatty acids are needed in our body, but when they are not in balance with omega-3s (the most often recommended ratio being 2:1) they can actually increase the occurrence of cardiovascular disease, diabetes, arthritis, cancer, Alzheimer's disease, and weight gain. To reduce this undesirable effect, severely limit the consumption of processed and fast foods, the use of the unsuitable oils, regular mayonnaise, commercial salad dressings (all high in omega-6 fatty acids), and focus on the intake of omega-3 foods.

Almonds, pecans, cashews, peanuts, hazel, pine and Brazil nuts, sesame, sunflower and pumpkin seeds have proportionately higher content of omega-6 to omega-3 fatty acids but have other health benefits so use them, but have more of the omega-3 rich variety.

Soak nuts and seeds in water overnight. Use a glass or ceramic container with a lid and store in the refrigerator. If you are pressed for time, soak nuts and seeds for minimum of twenty minutes or at least rinse under running water. Soaking improves the flavor and increases the enzyme activity, therefore the nutritional value and digestibility.

Do not drink icy cold liquids during or right after a meal. The stomach has to work hard to restore normal body temperature which causes you to loose energy. Also, if the meal contains a considerable amount of fat, the cold environment congeals fats so they cling as unwanted deposits to the digestive tract walls.

It is a good practice to skim off any fat floating on top of your soups, gravies, stews, and stocks.

Almond, coconut, goat, and rice milks are easier to digest than cow's milk. Scalding cow's milk may improve its digestion. The natural calcium content in cow's milk is higher than in the non-dairy milks but most of these milks are calcium fortified. Make sure that you shake the fortified milk well before using because calcium has the tendency to settle to the bottom of the container. Do not rely only on this source for your total calcium supply.

A whole egg (preferably free-range) is very nutritious. You don't have to be afraid of its cholesterol content. Actually, it is the ratio between the LDLs and HDLs that is important to consider. In an egg, the ratio is in favor of the desirable HDLs that help sweep away fatty particles so they do not adhere to blood vessels' walls and clog them. We can be grateful to nature for this great product. If you consume the suggested daily allotment of fruit, vegetables, and whole grains, you can enjoy one egg a day.

According to some studies, the free-range egg contains more beta-carotene (the precursor of vitamin A) and lutein, both important for the health of the eyes; the pronounced orange color of the free-range egg yolk versus the pale yellow of the commercial yolk attests to this finding. More omega-3 fatty acids, vitamins E and D, and less of the saturated fat were also found in the eggs of freely running birds than in the eggs of hens kept in tight factory quarters. On the other hand, some studies report no significant difference as to the nutritive values between factory (commercial) and free-range eggs. The choice is yours.

Iron supplementation may be necessary in case of blood loss during surgical procedures. Iron is best taken with food to prevent upset stomach. It is best absorbed and utilized in the presence of vitamin C. Be sure to eat an orange, kiwi, papaya, strawberries, bell peppers, vitamin C fortified juice, or take a vitamin C supplement with iron.

Constipation can be caused by some medications (codeine, iron), lack of fluids, fiber, motion, regular eating habits, or all of the above. The primary task of the large intestine is to conserve (reabsorb) water. Inadequate or slow peristalsis, wave-like movements of the intestines, cause waste products to stay in the large intestine longer, and become harder, because more water is reabsorbed over longer period of time, resulting in constipation.

Some foods (whole grain products, dried fruits, fresh fruits, vegetables, legumes) leave many indigestible particles that effectively stimulate the intestinal walls to move faster. Fats, buttermilk, yogurt, honey, and fish have directly stimulating properties. Gastrointestinal emptying is slowed by strong tea, cocoa, chocolate, white rice, white flour products, cheese, red wine, and some medications and supplements.

Even though the intestines should be stimulated, they should not be mechanically overloaded. For instance, too much fiber in form of fiber supplements could impair the utilization of electrolytes (sodium, potassium, magnesium, etc.). These would be flushed out prematurely, depriving the body of the necessary nutrients. Moderation is the answer; start with half of the manufacturer suggested dosage and drink a full glass of water each time.

Reducing diets can also bring on constipation due to the decreased amount of the 'propellers': sugars and fats. This can be corrected by increased intake of fluids, vegetables, fruits, and whole grain products, and also by exercise.

Before turning to commercial laxatives, try drinking a glass (8oz/ 250ml) of lukewarm water in the morning on an empty stomach. If that is not a sufficient remedy, ingest half a glass of prune juice or 1 cup of plain yogurt or buttermilk blended with four figs, dates, or one cup of blueberries. If necessary, carefully repeat at bedtime. A word of caution: under no circumstances take a laxative and a sleeping pill at the same time. There may be other reasons for constipation, so consult your physician if dietary measures fail.

> *'Doctor' complains a patient, 'I have difficulty concentrating. I am thinking about a thousand things at once.'*
>
> *'Take two cups of buttermilk every day,' advises the physician.*
>
> *'Buttermilk?' queries the patient.*
>
> *'Absolutely; in a while you will be thinking of one thing only!'*

Do not panic if you see discolored stools or urine. First consider whether you ate any red beets, blueberries, blackberries, or spinach the previous day. Some medications may also alter the color of stools or urine. For example, iron supplements darken stools, and B vitamins turn urine bright yellow. Conversely, black, tarry stools or visible blood should be immediately reported to your physician.

Diarrhea is the uncomfortable race in which the runner may be overrun. Nevertheless, a short bout of diarrhea is less problematic than longstanding constipation. Sure, one may feel as energetic as the limp tail of a dog, but eventually this will pass. Diarrhea is usually caused by sensitivities to food, the wrong combination of foods (and drinks), new medications or supplements, overexposure to sun, and bacteria. There are also more serious medical reasons for diarrhea, but our focus is on the basic ones.

It is usually best to let diarrhea run its course (no pun intended). The body is getting rid of an irritant thus cleansing itself before the repair can begin. Therefore, if you have the comfort of a nearby washroom, do not have to travel, or go to work, cooperate for a day with the wisdom of the body and do not take any binding potions. If diarrhea is severe, or persists after 24 hours, consult your physician.

The main concern is to compensate for fluid and electrolytes loss. Drink at least 2 liters (8 cups) of liquid or more per day to prevent dehydration sometimes manifested by dizziness. Start with black, green or camomile tea. Soda crackers, white toast, banana, white rice, consomme, and applesauce can be added next. Ingest a small amount every hour or more often. If you tolerate yogurt, acidophilus milk, or kefir, then introduce these slowly to your diet; they are good sources of probiotic factors restoring the depleted beneficial bacteria in the digestive tract (refer to the information about antibiotics). Probiotics can also be taken as supplements in capsules.

Some people are sensitive to vitamin C. If you take more than 1,000mg a day and get diarrhea, reduce the dose to regulate the bowel movement.

Stay away from fatty and fried foods, dairy products (with the exception of the above mentioned probiotic items), spicy dishes, fresh fruit (with the exception of bananas), meat, alcohol, and artificial sweeteners (with the exception of stevia) for couple days. Be careful with coffee, since it may irritate the digestive system.

Abdominal distention caused by flatulence (gas) is another unpleasant condition where certain food may be the main culprit. Beware of gas forming foods such as cauliflower, broccoli (less offensive if only the crowns are used), kale, onion, garlic (the last two particularly if used fresh), radishes, pulses (lentils, beans, peas, chickpeas), pears, apples, peaches, blueberries, cherries, melons. Milk, sugar, and fatty foods are also on the list for sensitive digestive systems.

Write down what you eat and drink for several days and notice the correlation between the symptoms and the items you ingested. By identifying the pattern, it is then easier to deal with the troublemakers.

To alleviate flatulence, eat slowly, chew thoroughly. Eat apples and pears peeled, stewed, or baked. Eat fruit before meals on an empty stomach. Drink before eating fruit, especially with pits. For instance, drinking water after consuming cherries can produce wicked gas that even the Goodyear blimp would envy. Soak beans overnight, drain, add fresh water, and cook till tender.

Drink teas made from fennel, anise, caraway seed, peppermint, camomile, or ginger. Pour 1 cup of boiling water over one to two teaspoons of the spice, herb, or several slices of fresh ginger root, let steep for 10 minutes. Peppermint is great but don't drink it just before lying down or bedtime — it could cause heartburn.

Beano, Swedish bitters, broad spectrum digestive enzymes, and simethicone (Gas X, Ovol) are just a few of the products that can also come to the rescue.

Exercising your way to greater strength and flexibility

Why do you need to exercise? Movement enhances blood flow to the tissues which brings the nourishment needed for healing. Motion also improves health by increasing flexibility, strength, stamina, and muscle tone. If possible, practice the suggested exercises before your hospitalization so that when needed, you will be able to perform them easily, almost automatically.

Breathing exercises are especially important. Anyone receiving a general anesthetic will be urged to clear their lungs as soon as possible to avoid any complications. The respiratory technician and the nurse will take care of you, but if you know how to help yourself and proceed on your own, you will recover from the effect of the anesthetic much faster.

The breathing exercises not only ventilate your lungs, but they can also effectively calm and relax you. One is not exempt from occasional moments of anxiety, no matter how cool, calm, and collected. A tense reaction to an unknown situation may surprise you, and if not checked at its onset, may develop into a more gripping state of anxiety, hampering normal body functions.

The diaphragm, the muscle separating the lungs from the abdominal organs, is the point of focus during the breathing exercise. When done correctly, the exercise will help regulate the heartbeat, open up the lungs for greater oxygen intake, increase circulation to the major organs, and relax you.

You can do this exercise lying down, sitting, or even walking. For the most effective breathing, take a deep breath through the nose, distend the lower part of the rib cage (try to appear very pregnant), and fill the chest with air. Hold the breath for a moment, and then, slowly exhale through the mouth, as if blowing out a candle. At the same time, suck in the stomach. It may seem unnatural at first, but with practice, it will feel normal.

Adjust the rhythm of inhalation and exhalation according to your comfort. The exhalation should be slightly longer than the inhalation. To establish the rhythm, count silently: inhale (one), hold (one), exhale (one, two, three). With practice, you can prolong each count. Do ten repetitions as often as you can, at least once every waking hour.

After the breathing exercise, you may experience an urge to cough; do not suppress it. Have a pillow handy in case you have an incision in the chest, or abdominal area, and press the pillow firmly against the incision for the duration of the cough. Bring up any phlegm, and spit it out. Do not swallow it! Have a tissue within easy reach.

To counteract anxiety, here is an alternative exercise. As soon as you start feeling uneasy, breathe deeply in whatever way you find comfortable and concentrate on counting down from 10 or 20. In your mind's eye, see the numbers being written on a blackboard, one by one, in roman and arabic numerals (XV, 15; XIV, 14; XIII, 13; etc.). This will take your mind off the upsetting thoughts and give you time to calm yourself.

Practice the following simple exercises unless otherwise indicated by hospital staff.

Start your morning exercise with 1, 2, 3 up, then 1, 2, 3, down — now the other eyelid.

Just joking, now seriously:

Stretch your neck to either side, press the back of your head against the bed or the headrest of the armchair, if you are sitting. Do not clench your teeth, relax the jaw.

Move your fingers as if playing an imaginary piano, make fists, circle your hands (but not the one with the I.V.).

Lying on your back, move your toes; dig them into the bed, then relax. Circle your feet.

With the foot flat on the bed, slide it up bending the knee, then slide it back down. Exercise the other leg the same way. Repeat at least ten times every hour. It is very important to move your legs to increase circulation, prevent stagnation of blood and formation of blood clots.

Sitting on the bed or chair, straighten one leg at a time, lift it up one foot off the ground, and point the toes to the ceiling. Hold this position to the count of ten, and then put the leg down. Repeat five times with each leg.

Before getting up and walking, sit on the edge of the bed for a couple minutes, move your legs, put on safe footwear, and slowly get into the upright position. Be sure to have proper support and assistance for the first few times to prevent falls.

Whenever standing for any length of time, don't just stand with your feet planted. Promote circulation by shifting your weight from one foot to the other.

One of the most effective exercises is simply walking with the arms swinging rhythmically. Start slowly, gradually, and cautiously. Support yourself with a walker, cane, or crutches, and ask for help, if necessary. Be conscious of your posture. Do not hunch forward in an attempt to protect an incision. This is a common mistake. Straighten up, press the shoulder blades back and together. This will prevent adhesions and the scar will become more flexible, less puckered. By stretching your chest you will also ventilate the lungs better.

Once back home, walking in fresh air in nature would be ideal. Deep breathing delivers the oxygen to your blood cells more efficiently. With enhanced circulation, the organs obtain essential nutrients more readily, and the metabolism gets a boost. Being in nature induces deeper relaxation and instills a sense of order and belonging. Do not give up on walking if a park, beach, meadow, or forest are not in the vicinity, or if the weather is inclement. Create a walking corridor anywhere, even if it is just a few meters long — in your room, the hallway, a mall: walk, walk, walk.

To improve alignment of hips and spine, place a pillow between your knees when lying on your side. While resting on your back, place a pillow under your thighs (between the buttocks and knees).

To prevent or relieve a stiff neck, either sitting or standing, turn your head to the right, and nod gently up and down several times. Repeat on the left. Place a rolled up towel under your neck when lying on your back or side to maintain proper alignment.

If your hands or fingers get numb, particularly when lying down, insert a small pillow under the armpit, and make sure the wrist is neither bent nor flexed. Move the fingers, circle the hand, make a fist, and then relax.

To relax stiff shoulders, stand next to a table, or a stable chair, and support yourself by one arm. Bend over slightly and swing the other arm back and forth freely, like a pendulum, 15 to 20 times. Circle the arm gently clockwise and counterclockwise 15 to 20 times in each direction. Switch sides, and relax the other arm in the same fashion.

To strengthen the legs and thighs, stand with your back touching the wall, legs planted shoulder width apart and feet flat on the ground. Slide down and up several times, progressively lower.

When lifting an object from the ground, squat as much as you can, reach for the object while arching your back, and then slowly straighten up holding the object centrally close to your body.

For support while walking, use two walking poles, rather than one, so that your joints are equally supported, neither side is taxed more than the other, and the exercise is more efficient, engaging not only your legs but your arms as well.

If you have to sit or stand for a long time, move your feet and legs often, as described earlier.

Smile!

Include one more simple exercise
that positively affects all and satisfies:
a sincere smile goes a long way
to brighten every person's day.
Only a fleeting second it will take,
but big barriers it will break.

As soon as you smile, a positive contact is established, even with a total stranger. This invitation to kindness is hard to ignore even by the grouchiest person. A genuine smile with kind intention shows appreciation for life, and the eyes, the windows of the soul, reflect and project this inner charge.

Every day, life gives plenty of chances to respond with kindness. You may restrain yourself from making an impatient gesture, a disapproving frown, or an unkind remark. Instead, give praise and express gratitude for help, care, and time received. Accompanied by a smile, your positive conduct will shine through even more.

> **PEST**: "The full range of my talents is available to psyche you up to practice what you have learned. So now, add a smile, and let's get to work.
>
> "Inhale through the nose expanding the belly like a big balloon, hold your breath, hold, hold,

now blow out a hundred imaginary candles. Blow hard. Try again. This is the sequence: nose, balloon, candles. Ready, go! Breathe in, let me hear the air rush through your nose. Don't forget to inflate the balloon, hold your breath, and then breathe it all out through your mouth. That was good.

"This breathing exercise will, hopefully, make you cough, and bring up some phlegm. Press a pillow or your hands against the incision to protect it. If coughing does not happen naturally, force yourself to cough. Bring up the phlegm, and spit it out. Way to go!

"Moving on, to prevent stiffness, stretch your neck from side to side several times. Now, push the back of your head into the pillow, keep your chin down, and hold this position for about five seconds. Relax. Repeat both exercises at least five times every waking hour.

"How about playing the piano? Do the full scales, not just chop sticks with two fingers. All your fingers have to run nimbly over the keyboard. That's the way. Keep the circulation going. Make a fist, squeeze hard, and then relax. Play some more, I'm all ears. Squeeze again. Relax.

"Now, let's concentrate on your legs and feet. Send them appreciative thoughts, and give them tender loving care. Don't grant clots a free cruise in sluggish blood vessels. To stimulate the blood flow, wiggle the toes, dig them into the bed, circle your feet, rock them from toe to heel, bend your knees, do whatever you want, just don't let your lower limbs lie dormant for a long time. Keep going; repeat each motion at least ten times every hour. Think of your circulation as a fast freeway, not a congested one-way street during rush hour. You want to get home as fast and safely as possible.

"You are doing well, give yourself a pat on the shoulder. I'll give you a breather now, and when you are ready, we'll walk.

The physician is assessing Harry's mental sharpness.

'Conjugate the verb "to walk" in simple present, Harry.'

'I walk, you walk...'

'Faster, Harry, if you please!' the doctor urges.

'I run, you run...' obliges Harry.

"I am back. Before walking, do a mental warm up first. Recall the importance of exercising, see yourself stronger with each effort, healing faster, and feeling happy with the result. Affirm, 'Every day, in every way, I am getting better and better.' Feel it in the core of your being.

"What is the first thing you have to do in preparation for walking? Make sure your johnny shirt is tied? That's true, but what I mean is, move to the edge of the bed, swing your legs down, and sit there for a while. Good. Next, lift one leg at a time, point the toes to the ceiling, and hold this position while counting to ten.

"Now, plant your feet on the ground, and walk slowly. Straighten up, put the shoulder blades together, don't slump, suck in the stomach, stick out your hips, expand the chest, and breathe deeply. Too much to remember? All right, I'll make it easier. Pretend you are a model walking on a runway. So, lights, camera, smile, and walk!

"Did you say something about a slave driver? I may be a little demanding, but in my defense, I recognize all your dormant potential, so I know that I am not overtaxing you. I realize that you may feel a little tired, but trust me, you do have enough energy — just apply your will and use it. You will be pleasantly surprised at how able you are, what means you possess, and what progress you are making. I am proud of your every effort, and your success and satisfaction are also my reward.

"That does not mean you can now rest on your laurels, or your behind. Get back to work. Walk, walk, walk!"

Attending to mind and spirit

Just as our advice on nutrition is not a comprehensive work in that field, by the same token we are not offering a deep plunge into the mysteries of the mind and spirit. We are suggesting some simple but potent methods to calm the mind, and consequently, relax the body, two very important elements in recovery. These exercises can also be used as a springboard for other practices aimed at increasing spiritual awareness.

When speaking of body, mind, spirit, and soul, we are not suggesting that the following explanation is the only valid way to perceive these aspects of our being. Rather, we are defining a concept used within the framework of our book, as we, through longstanding interest and resourcing, can best understand and present.

The body/ mind organism is a vessel through which the spirit expresses itself on the material plane of existence. The spirit, which endows this organism with creative inspiration above and beyond the body/mind processes, has its origin in the infinite spirit, the limitless source of everything that exists. This vital source (the God-force) permeates and unites all aspects of life. It is ultimate love; unconditionally giving, uplifting, creating, guiding, and lighting the way to all encompassing progress. We envision our soul as the Spirit enriched entity, a pool of energies corresponding to our aspirations, perceptions, intentions, deeds, values, ideals, and their realizations.

The influence of the mind (positive and negative) on the state of health is widely recognized. Every part of your being — from the many facets of the "I" identity to the infinitesimal structure of a cell — has its own awareness, its own consciousness. The energy of your thoughts and beliefs, your responses to people and situations produce reactions and affect the consciousness, demonstrating the law of cause and effect.

All components of your being — body, mind, and spirit — are interconnected and affect one another. The concept of the relaxation response has been well known for millennia. In 1960 Dr. Herbert Benson started scientific research in this field. Since then, numerous studies confirmed that when brain activity is quieted by praying, meditating, regulated breathing, playing music, practicing yoga, or any other activity requiring calming concentration, positive changes are induced in the body. Antioxidant and anti-inflammatory processes are stimulated. Heart rate, blood pressure, asthma, skin diseases, digestive problems, anxiety, depression, insomnia, and many other conditions can be improved.

Devoting 15 to 20 minutes daily to some form of relaxation will greatly benefit not only the body and speed up your recovery, but also bring about more harmonious and balanced state of the entire being. Choose a method that is comfortable and for which you feel an affinity. Attract the desired outcome by way of optimistic, trusting, uplifting, positive goal-oriented images, and affirmations. Do not evaluate the effort each time, just do it. Relax.

No amount of energy put into this practice is ever wasted. Perseverance and good intention are the keys that can gradually unlock the gateway to better understanding yourself and the purpose of life, the fulfilling of your needs, and the aspirations of the soul.

Ralph Waldo Emerson said, "We are all inventors, each sailing on a voyage of discovery, guided by a private chart of which there is no duplicate. The world is all gates, all opportunities."

Through your life journey, you will become increasingly aware of many guiding prompts and uncanny synchronicity of events: people you meet, books you read, places you visit, movies you see, music you hear, or a message you suddenly understand. All of this is provided to help your progress.

Find your own sign posts and follow their lead as time goes by. Our needs change and we too have to be flexible, adjusting to our inner promptings. Explore new concepts, widen your horizons, and get a closer look at your personal values and motives.

At different times, some ideas or concepts will strike the right chord with you while others may not. There is a right time for everything. If not today, then later, when the time is right you will happily respond to all nudges to quench your thirst for truth. With objectivity and tolerance you will be more and more receptive to the revelations of your true identity, your higher self.

Look for the good in others; experience the peaceful impact of forgiveness. It may take time to liberate yourself from the perception of unjust hurtful conduct, but persevere. Heartfelt forgiveness starts a positive chain reaction, leads to a peaceful mind, relaxed body, and ultimately a jubilant soul, and spirit.

Mentally create images of beauty, order, peace, and love whenever possible. They nourish the soul, inspire the mind, and strengthen the body. Saint Paul advises, "Whatever is true, whatever is honorable, whatever is just, whatever is pure, whatever is lovely, whatever is gracious, if there is any excellence, if there is anything worthy of praise, think about these things." Thought, like a magnet, readily attracts to its substance corresponding energies, so let your positive, kind thoughts work to your advantage.

Exercise #1

Focus on the source of your spiritual inspiration. Charge your breath with the qualities of that source and surrender to it with all humility. Inhale deeply and follow the same rhythm as in the breathing exercises. Exhale, and send this purified energy from the abdomen to your thighs, legs, feet, and toes. Repeat several times.

Next, when you exhale, send the energy to your heart, upper limbs, throat, and head. Repeat several times. If that seems like too much 'territory' to cover during one exhalation, split the cycle. After energizing the lower extremities, send the breath energy first to your shoulders, arms, hands, and fingers several times, and then to the heart, neck, and head. At the end of the exercise, give thanks.

Exercise #2

Breathe deeply and feel the flow of purity (an image of light, love, a healing fountain) enter your head and cascade down your neck, shoulders, arms, and hands to your finger tips. Continue with the same image, guiding the energy to your torso, legs, feet, toes, and into the ground. Visualize the washing away of tension and negative emotions, leaving you cleansed and peaceful, filled with whatever is presently needed. Say, "Thank you."

Exercise #3

If pressed for time, inhale and say to yourself, "I am gratefully receiving." Feel the loving energy of the source engulfing you, filling your whole being. Exhaling, say to yourself, "I am giving," and send as much kindness and love as you can envision out into space.

Do not dictate whom or what it should affect. Everything is connected and it will reach all. Offer your thanks.

Exercise #4

Picture yourself in a beautiful garden. Flowers, shrubs, and trees of your choice surround you. Focus on your favorite flower; notice the petals, the texture, the aroma, and the shades of colors. Look around, admire the majestic trees, the sun's rays penetrating their crowns, and shining on the path which makes its way through the velvety green grass. Hear birds chirping, a woodpecker pecking, a brook trickling and bubbling over pebbles and rocks, tall grass moving with the wind. See a squirrel munching on an acorn, and then jumping from branch to branch in an oak tree.

You are alone but not lonely, connected with nature, a part of the universal order you trust. Surrender to it. Become aware of the divine within you, your true identity. Now perceive it as a brilliant, vibrating, penetrating, beautiful light. The light is charged with everything dear to your heart, every value you uphold: beauty, order, peace, forgiveness, joy, friendship, understanding, tolerance, and most of all, unconditional love. Open yourself, accept, and absorb this energy.

Allow the light to fill your entire being, give you strength, and the certainty of being cared for and loved. Let it heal negative memories, melt away all tension and worries, fill you with everything you need.

All is well. You know that you are never alone and with that knowledge comes peace. Repeat to yourself, "All is well." If it is in accordance with your personal belief, affirm, "Wherever I am, God (the infinite loving source) is. I am in God. God is in me." Express your gratitude.

> **PEST**: "As you well know, you cannot always control life's happenings; however, your perception and reaction to them is completely in your power. Try to look at all situations in an

objective, tolerant, and kind manner. This starts a positive chain reaction for the benefit of all.

A psychologist, lecturing an audience, holds up a glass. Everyone is expecting the usual question about the glass of water perceived either half empty or half full. Instead, the lecturer surprises them by asking, 'How heavy is the glass?' She then explains, 'The weight depends on how long I hold the glass. After a minute, I hardly feel the weight. After one hour, I will find it quite heavy, my arm will ache. After holding it all day, my arm will feel paralyzed. The glass still weighs the same, but the longer I hold it, the heavier it will seem. Stress and worries are like that glass; when you think about them for a little while, nothing happens. Dwelling on them longer will make you feel uncomfortable. Thinking about a problem all day, will hurt and immobilize you, and keep you from concentrating on anything else. So, make sure you put the glass away in time, don't carry it all day long, and, especially, don't bring it to bed at night.'

"To apply this analogy practically, acknowledge any troubling thought as soon as it starts. Even if you cannot specifically identify the source of your momentary anxiety, begin a deep breathing exercise. In addition, you may also count backwards, repeat a meaningful word or sentence, concentrate on your spiritual source, or use an uplifting visualization — whatever relaxes you best. This way, you stop any negative input before it germinates and grows. Instead, you begin to restore your balance.

"You are now better able to identify and resolve the actual problem by perceiving the issue more objectively. What is troubling you? Put aside any initial negative reaction. Look at the problem from the higher spiritual perspective. What may seem like a threat, may actually be an opportunity to unveil a needed change, a chance for improvement, and a new positive approach, beneficial to all. Call the next process a challenge. Concentrating on one step at a time, outline a plan to resolve whatever is troubling you, but do not 'hold the glass too long.' Put your plan into action, observe the results, and adjust the plan as necessary.

"If your problem solving involves interacting with another individual, approach it with an open mind, patience, and tolerance. Even if the issue is not immediately rectified, keep wishing the other party well, and concentrate on other tasks. If deep-seated negative emotions remain persistently difficult to resolve, seek professional help.

"The infinite source of all that exists reaches out to you, constantly offering love, solace, and help. When you connect with this source, your heart opens to compassion for yourself and your fellow beings. Bring this aspect of spiritual nurturing to awareness as often as you can. You are part of the Oneness. Invoke the generous, inexhaustible source of abundance, receive and cherish its gifts with gratitude, and share them selflessly with others."

Recuperating at home

Once you return home, you will progressively take on more responsibility for your needs. Proper nutrition, exercise, and relaxation are the paramount concerns. Please review the previous advice on these topics and apply it as faithfully as you are able.

Whether we study the concepts of twelth century mystics, or contemporary physicists, the idea of "each part being in the whole and the whole being in each part" is a recurrent belief. Everything that we, as mankind, have experienced is stored in each of us, just as our instincts, reactions, emotional charges, values, behaviors, and deeds are now streaming into that vast pool of knowledge. Whatever our ancestors sowed, we are reaping. Whatever we sow presently will form the future.

Helping each other is one of the major factors contributing to personal growth. People become involved for various reasons; some may be self-oriented, others partially or totally altruistic. Many times it seems to be easier to offer help than to receive it. All of us have to learn not only to give, but also to accept service with love.

"I don't want to be a burden to my family" is a frequently expressed concern. Since your life is interwoven with the lives of others for a reason, you may never know why it is important to be in someone's presence. By simply being, you may be giving another person an opportunity to do a good deed, learn from you, or enrich themselves by serving you. The person who accepts the service learns to be humble, trusting, and thankful. The one who serves, learns to be patient, tolerant, respectful, and generous. Thus both the giver and the receiver contribute positively to the collective consciousness.

All forms of energy (food, thoughts, air, sunshine, exercise) produce certain outcomes; this is the law of **cause and effect, action and reaction.** For instance, consistently healthy food intake, and a relaxed, positively charged state of mind (**cause/ action**) supply you with the elements needed not only for proper functioning and healing, but also for self-realization, pleasure, and contribution to the greater good (**effect/ reaction**).

Conversely, unhealthy eating habits, negative images, anxiety, fear, pessimistic outlook, or any other stress (**cause/ action**) can not only impair proper function of the digestive organs, but also result in lack of energy, and zest for life (**effect/ reaction**). When you do not feel well physically and mentally (**cause/action**), you are not as able to recover readily, enjoy life fully, or focus on needs of others (**effect/reaction**).

Please, be selective at all times with your input whether eating, reading, observing, or participating in social activities. Avoid violence, anger, malice, fear, or any other negative stimuli that could leave an unhealthy imprint on your physical, mental, and spiritual being, and slow your recovery. Nourish yourself with positively inspired ideas, books, music, and art. Surround yourself by optimistic, like-minded fellow beings, wish everyone well, and perform good deeds whenever possible. Everything connects on a small and large scale. Once we acknowledge that every individual influences the course of human development and growth, then the importance of good intentions and actions becomes obvious. Let us try to contribute to this positive chain reaction.

PEST: "Aren't you glad to be home? Welcome back, and let's get to work. There is a lot to do and your ever-present **PEST** is eager to help to restore you to better health. You need optimal nutrition, sleep, activity, and relaxation.

"You may not have been enthusiastic about your hospital venture, but be gracious and acknowledge that without the professional care, your health would have suffered. Now you have a brighter future ahead. The medical procedure is history, your appetite is slowly returning, and you can cater to your needs through a routine that suits you...to a point, because I have some suggestions as well. Consider my

Poetic Appetizer

Eat slowly, chew well,
don't gulp big chunks of food,
enjoy, give thanks,
proceed in a cheerful mood.
While eating,
no books, TV, browsing the Internet,
appreciate the blessings
of your daily bread instead.
Cultivate these seeds of care
to provide a healing atmosphere.

"It is not only what you eat, but how you eat it. Enjoy your meal in peace, rest briefly, and then be ready to move again. Follow this golden rule: rest, activity, rest, activity. There is a saying that goes, 'take it easy, but take it.' Embrace this concept.

"Rest means relaxation, not having a snooze whenever you start to yawn. An occasional nap is fine, but save most of the sleeping for nighttime. Relax with a good book, engage in a stimulating or fun conversation, do a relaxation routine, or sit outdoors in fresh air and sunshine. Since laughter is good medicine, make sure you get a good dose every day. Develop a refreshing sense of humor, laugh with a friend, or even at yourself.

A 50 year old patient, having just completed a physical check-up and hinting for a compliment, remarks:

'People tell me all the time that I don't look my age. What would you say, doctor?' '

Absolutely,' responds the physician, 'you don't look a day over 65...'

"Smiling and laughing will help you overcome trying situations, live in the present moment optimistically, and climb the wellness ladder more easily. Someone said, 'If life gives you a hundred reasons to cry, keep acknowledging a thousand reasons to smile.'

The Way To Health

If you eat well, not on the run,
rest, and frolic, and have some fun,
stretch your body and exercise,
then wellness will be your prize.
To give a fresh start to your day,
let relaxation lead the way.
When harmony is your intent,
the effort will pay dividend.
Be positive in your approach,
let the good spirit be your coach!"

Promoting good sleeping habits

Sleep is vital. While you are sleeping, your whole being is resting, healing, energizing, and preparing for the next waking cycle without any conscious input from you. Our ancestors noticed that sleep before midnight provides greater recuperative and restorative powers than sleep after midnight. Today, sleep experts support this observation.

- To best induce regular deep sleep, follow the same routine every night to establish a pattern.
- Go to bed at the same time well before midnight.
- Do not eat a large, hard to digest, or spicy meal at suppertime.
- Have your snack no later than an hour before bedtime.
- Don't drink any alcohol for a couple of hours before bedtime.
- Enjoy caffeine-free soothing herbal teas like camomile, lemon balm, passion- flower, or sleepy time blend.
- Drink most of the required fluids during the day to prevent numerous night- time excursions to the bathroom.

- Avoid any strenuous activities at least one hour before bedtime.

- Choose something uplifting, humorous, and relaxing to watch or read.

In Shakespeare's time, the mattress was secured on bed frames by ropes which could be pulled to adjust the firmness. The phrase, 'Goodnight, sleep tight,' probably originated then, and was used by well-wishers convinced that a firm mattress guarantees a good night's rest. Is your mattress comfortably supportive?

Take calcium with magnesium and/ or L-tryptophan, an amino acid, to aid relaxation and regulate sleep. Remember the old remedy of drinking a glass of warm milk with honey? This works because milk contains calcium and L-tryptophan. The latter is also found in honey, bananas, black cherries, nuts, seeds, oats, legumes, and poultry. Based on this finding, here is a selection of some suitable bedtime snacks: home made granola (recipe section) with milk and banana slices, oatmeal porridge with nuts and honey, a handful of cherries, or a small glass of pure cherry juice, cheese and whole grain crackers, yogurt smoothie with hemp and honey, whole grain toast with nut butter and honey.

There are many pharmaceutical, prescription, and alternative medicine sleep aids available. Before resorting to any of these products, please consult the appropriate medical professional.

Fear, anxiety, worries, and stress can play havoc with sleep. You toss and turn, imagine situations far more threatening in your thoughts than in reality, and foster negative emotions. In the words of a French proverb, 'Some of your griefs you have cured and the sharpest you have survived, but what torments of pain you endured from evils that never arrived!'

Fear (False Evidence Appearing Real) has no shape, no form, and no power. It is nothing until you create its image and give it power. We cannot completely avoid negative thoughts, but we have the ability to control our reactions to them. Stop the fear in the beginning before it develops into a major fantasy. When an unpleasant thought appears, acknowledge it, accept its existence, but then push it gently away. Do a short relaxation routine, and focus on a pleasant image.

As part of your bedtime routine, a couple minutes of deep breathing, playing a disc with a calming theme, a short prayer, repetition of a short sentence or a meaningful word (mantra), will help to relax you.

PEST: "Allow me a little bedtime humor:

'Did you know that sleep is the best beautifying tool?'

'Really? I guess, that's why I like to sleep so much!'

"Peaceful images open the gateways to relaxation. Create your own, or feel free to use my suggestions.

- Feel the peace of a starry night with the moonlight reflecting on the calm waters of a lake. Hear the loon, crickets, and frogs.

- Witness the sunrise or sunset over the mountaintops, or over the sea.

- Walk into a beautiful fountain of healing, loving, purifying (divine) light.

- Envision a tree dressed in magnificent array of various seasons.

- Visualize yourself on a mountain top. Admire the range of majestic mountains in the hazy colors of a fresh morning.

- Hear the cowbells from the valley, and picture lush meadows flooded with wild flowers.

- Follow a butterfly or a bee flying from blossom to blossom.

- Feed the birds and chipmunks.

- Fly with an eagle.

- Feel a loving hand caressing your forehead, soothing and relaxing.

- Think peace and loving care; surrender to it, and let go of everything else.

Good night."

Assisting the patient before, during, and after hospitalization

This chapter is addressed to family members, friends, and all persons wishing to extend a helpful hand to a patient. The material is divided into three parts: for the period before admission, during, and after hospitalization. Naturally, some tasks mentioned in the preparation stage may be repeated during the patient's recuperation. If possible, read the whole book to increase the scope and effectiveness of your assistance.

You will undoubtedly come up with a variety of other possibilities than the following suggestions. The level of your involvement will depend on the amount of time you can spend and what task you choose to do. Keep in mind that no good deed is ever too small and will always be appreciated.

Please, stay away from the patient if you have any infectious disease like a cold or flu. You can give your support instead by calling, texting, Skyping, and arranging any needed services without direct contact.

If your presence is necessary, observe hygienic measures rigorously to reduce the patient's exposure to any germs. Wash your hands frequently with soap and water for at least 15 seconds each time, particularly before handing things to the patient. Wear a surgical mask and gloves; change your clothing often, or use a gown; do not share the patient's food, dishes, and utensils; do not kiss or hug the patient, and generally keep as much distance as possible.

To speed up your own recovery, take good care of yourself following the advice presented in this book. Even when you are healthy, incorporate the hygienic measures into your daily routine for your own and the patient's benefit.

Before admission

Read the chapter 'Preparing for Hospitalization' and offer to assist the patient with the following tasks:

- Discuss and obtain the chosen preventative supplements suggested in the above-mentioned chapter.

- Accompany the patient to pre-admission medical appointments, procedures, tests, and clinics.

- Transport the patient wherever necessary.

- Obtain home health care products and equipment (crutches, walker, hand bars, adjustable toilet seat, bath chair), and install them if necessary.

- Encourage the patient to practice deep breathing, relaxation, visualization, and exercise routines.

- Arrange caregivers' services, meal delivery, pet and plant care, and mail pick up.

- Perform household chores.

- Stock up groceries.

- Prepare and freeze single servings meals.

- Pack the suitcase for the hospital.
- Accompany the patient to the hospital, and if possible stay till he or she is admitted.

During hospitalization

Visiting the convalescent is a commendable act of care, but make sure the patient is up to it. Do not stay too long unless specifically asked, and watch for signs of tiredness. For everyone's comfort, speak in a low, soothing voice. Offer help when needed, for instance:

- Arrange necessary items so they are easily accessible.
- Position pillows to provide comfort.
- Bring fresh water.
- Help with meals (position the table, cut the portions, feed the patient).
- Fill the washbasin with warm water, so the bedridden patient can wash up before and after meals.
- Assist with oral hygiene.
- Refresh patient's face with a wet face cloth.
- Gently rub feet and hands if requested.
- Read to the patient.
- If the patient is ambulatory, suggest walking and accompany her/ him.
- Encourage breathing exercises. Lead by counting: breathe in (one), hold (one), breathe out (one, two, three).

- Promote good posture and the recommended exercises.

- Be alert for any signs of distress; call a nurse if necessary.

You may also consider preparing the patient's home for his/her return:

- Dust, sweep, clean the fridge, remove garbage, change the bedclothes, wash the laundry.

- Clear away any clutter, securing an obstacle-free passage for the patient's safety.

- Place essentials such as an alarm clock, flashlight, or battery-operated lamp, bottled water, spare blanket, facial tissues, and phone within the patient's easy reach.

- Plan and prepare a few meals, keeping in mind any special dietary requirements.

- Shop for groceries.

- Ask the patient's pharmacist to arrange for compliance packaging of medications and supplements (individualized single dose blister packing) if necessary.

Choosing appropriate gifts

Flowers are lovely, but consider the possibility of allergies of all people concerned. Also, there may not be enough room at the patient's bedside.

Please do not give chocolates. The patient's metabolism of sugar may be impaired, particularly after major surgery, due to glucose infusion, restricted food intake, and increased stress to the body. Any one or combination of these factors may be responsible for undesirably high blood sugar level. Adding concentrated sugar would exacerbate this condition. Chocolate can also cause constipation, an unwelcome irregularity especially at this time.

Suitable treats are nuts (if the patient has no allergies, or difficulty chewing), well washed fresh fruit, dried fruit, unsweetened fruit juices, apple sauce, juiced vegetables, multigrain baked (not fried) crackers, bottled water, homemade soups, granola, and pudding. You may want to bring gifts to entertain and lift the spirit, such as a small book, e-book, magazine, video game, music, etc.

After hospitalization

- At the hospital, gather all the patient's belongings and prescriptions with a medication schedule.

- Acquaint yourself with any instructions about the patient's care since he or she may be unable to fully absorb all the information.

- Accompany the patient and on the way home get the prescribed medications.

- Draw up a daily medication schedule (if not already provided by the hospital). Supervise that the patient takes the prescriptions correctly.

- At home, settle the patient comfortably, and make sure he/she is getting enough fluids (at least two liters a day); please, refer to the chapter on nutrition.

- Provide a variety of homemade food items such as breads, shakes, smoothies, cookies, fruit salads.

- Only when the patient's digestion and elimination return to normal, you may offer a small piece of chocolate (15 to 20 grams or ½ ounce) or a small handful of chocolate covered nuts, raisins, cranberries, blueberries, or cherries once a day. Dark chocolate (raw organic or containing at least 72% cocoa) is preferable to milk chocolate for its antioxidant properties.

- Assist the patient with personal hygiene.

- Encourage the patient to ask for help with any household tasks you would be willing to do.

- As soon as possible, encourage the patient to exercise and walk, and accompany him or her. Your presence gives the patient a feeling of security, and stimulates her/ him to do more than when left alone.

It is wonderful that you are helping the patient in any way possible, but remember that the patient has to gradually become more independent. Aim for this goal from the very beginning of your care and the overall result will be gratifying.

Closing thoughts

The recuperation period is over, but the maintenance of your health and wellbeing is just as important and ongoing.

For our earthly existence, we need energy. From the all-sustaining source, this energy is available to us as spirit-enlivened thought and matter. The subtle energy of thoughts manifests in all actions and, consequently, their outcome. Matter provides the elements (food, oxygen, sunshine, gravitational pull) necessary for our physical processes. We prosper when all components are utilized in a productive, complementary way.

Individual needs change and one has to be able to adjust to a variety of situations. In your continuing quest for wellness, honor your body's needs for proper nourishment, invigorating motion, relaxation, fresh air, and restful sleep. Strengthen your intentions for healthy living through positive thoughts with a firm belief in their realization. Guided by the spirit, seek and follow the high principles and ideals to fulfill your true life purpose.

In adverse situations, do not give in to negative emotions. Use the available spiritual, mental, and material tools to clear and grade the path for your power walk. Don't let the past limit your stride. Move on freely and optimistically.

In your life, there will be many opportunities for progressively greater understanding and fulfillment. Wherever your needs and aspirations take you, appreciate yourself, and offer loving kindness to all. Be well.

PEST: "You and I work well together, so let's keep the chat line open to share more in the future. Your symbolic ladder to wellness testifies to all that you have already accomplished. Some rungs are worn out more than others depending on how fast you climbed, fought for balance, or slipped and held on for dear life. There were even times when you thought you could go no further, but ultimately found the strength to continue.

"Your ladder has unlimited reach with extensions pointing in all directions, unfolding, and beckoning you to fulfill your potential. Be grateful for the opportunities, and pursue contentment, health, and inner harmony. Treat yourself and others with love, and with God's help, keep on keeping on."

ADDENDUM

Recipes

You may wonder whether these recipes are scrumptious or healthy. They can be both, depending on the ingredients you use. For instance, on the healthier end of the scale, when the recipe calls for flour, instead of using all-purpose flour, substitute spelt, kamut, quinoa, barley, whole wheat, rye, coconut, oat, or brown rice flour, or combine all-purpose flour with any of the above. Instead of cow's milk, use coconut, rice, or almond milk; instead of butter, use coconut butter, or combine both; instead of eggs (in case you are allergic, or otherwise concerned about their consumption), use egg replacer, ground flax seed, xanthan gum, tapioca, or arrowroot powder. Feel free to experiment.

Returning to the initial question, the words "healthy" and "scrumptious" may have different meanings for different people. Someone used to eating lots of the less healthy choices of nutrients, may not consider our creations delicious enough. On the opposite side of the spectrum, people who evaluate everything they consume from the ideal health point of view, may regard the recipes as not healthy enough. Our main goal is to provide reasonably healthy and affordable alternatives for most people, without deviating too far from their comfort zone during recuperation.

Hopefully, our good intentions will be well received. Enjoy!

Gusto Crepes

5 tablespoons flour
1 egg
½ cup milk
dash of salt
1 tablespoon honey
2 tablespoons coconut butter or grape seed oil for cooking

Makes 4 crepes.

1 crepe contains 3.5 g protein, 5.9 g fat, 10.7 g carbohydrates, and 111 calories.

Mix all ingredients till the batter is smooth. Heat the butter or oil in a frying pan. When sufficiently hot, pour 2 to 3 tablespoons of batter in the pan, spread it to the desired thickness, and slowly cook on both sides until lightly golden. (Before flipping, the top of the crepe should be dry).

The crepes can be made ahead of time and stored in the freezer (without the filling). They can be enjoyed as a desert filled with jam, fresh fruit, ice cream, light cream cheese mixed with grated lemon rind and honey, plain yogurt, or any combination of the above suggested items.

Strawberries and cream cheese filling for 4 crepes:

1 cup strawberries
2 tablespoons 15% light cream cheese
1 tablespoon honey, maple syrup, molasses, or agave syrup
grated lemon rind

1 crepe filling yields 1.87 g protein, 1.3 g fat, 7.7 g carbohydrates, and 47 calories.

As a savory dish (without honey in the batter), the crepes can be filled with cooked or fresh spinach, mixed vegetables, chicken, shrimp, salmon, mushrooms with onions, or any of your own creations.

The following is **the base used for all savory fillings**. Its nutrient and calorie count is included in each recipe.

2 teaspoons butter
2 teaspoons flour
1/4 cup milk
dash of salt
your favorite spices

In a small pan melt 2 teaspoons of butter, add 2 teaspoons of flour, stir for half a minute on low heat, add 1/4 cup of milk, and cook for 1 minute stirring constantly. Flavor with your favorite herbs or spices such as curry, marjoram, sage, basil, nutmeg, paprika, dill, etc. Add any above-mentioned savory items, spread over the crepes, roll or fold, and serve hot.

Poultry filling for 4 crepes:

Add to the base 60g (2 ounces) of cooked skinless poultry.

1 crepe filling yields 5.6 g protein, 3.05 g fat, 1.4 g carbohydrates, and 56 calories.

Salmon filling for 4 crepes:

Add to the base 60g (2 ounces) of cooked salmon.

1 crepe filling yields 5.16 g protein, 3.45 g fat, 1.4 g carbohydrates, and 57 calories.

Spinach filling for 4 crepes:

Add to the base:
1 cup cooked, finely chopped spinach
salt or 1/4 cube of Knorr bouillon
1 clove garlic
marjoram, sage, or rosemary
30g (1 ounce) 18% Swiss grated cheese — if desired

1 crepe filling without cheese yields 2.15 g protein, 2.80 g fat, 3.41 g carbohydrates, and 48 calories.
With cheese: 4.45 g protein, 4 g fat, 3.6 g carbohydrates, and 68 calories.

Mixed vegetables filling for 4 crepes:

Add to the base:
1 cup red peppers
1 cup broccoli
1/2 cup green or yellow beans
¼ cup onions
salt

All ingredients are steamed together until tender.
1 crepe filling yields 1.45 g protein, 2.5 g fat, 5.5 g carbohydrates, and 50 calories.

Mushroom filling for 4 crepes:

Add to the base:
3 cups washed, sliced mushrooms
1/2 cup onions
salt

All ingredients are steamed together until tender.
1 crepe filling yields 1.8 g protein, 0.15 g fat, 9 g carbohydrates, and 45 calories.

Fortifying Pulse Soup

Soak 1 cup of any of the pulses (lentils, beans, peas) overnight, then wash under running water and drain. Add 3 cups of fresh water or vegetable stock, any vegetables, if you wish, and cook until tender. (Canned lentils or beans may be used if pressed for time.) Add half a cube of vegetable bouillon, marjoram, a crushed garlic clove, and puree or liquefy with the cooked lentils in a blender. Dilute with stock or water according to your preference, and serve plain or with croutons. The soup freezes well.

Makes 4 portions.

1 portion contains 3.2 g proteins, 0.5 g fats, 4.5 g carbohydrates, and 35.5 calories.

Champion Mushroom Goulash

2 cups washed, sliced mushrooms
1/4 medium sliced onion
2 tsps coconut butter
1 clove garlic
2 tsps paprika
2 teaspoons flour
1/4 Knorr vegetable cube
1/2 cup coconut milk (or 10% cream if you tolerate dairy)

Makes 2 portions.

1 portion contains 3.7 g proteins, 10.4 g fats, 14.4 g carbohydrates, and 166 calories.

Melt the butter, add onion, and cook until almost transparent. Add mushrooms, Knorr cube, paprika, and crushed garlic; cover the bottom of the pan with water, and stew for 5 minutes. Sprinkle with flour, stir briefly, add milk, and cook till the mixture comes to boil.

The goulash may be served with rice, pasta, mashed potatoes, cooked pot barley, couscous, quinoa, or bread.

Two Goodies Soup

2 medium carrots
1/2 bunch asparagus
nutmeg, curry, or marjoram
2 cups vegetable stock or 1/2 cube Knorr vegetable bouillon with 2 cups water

Makes 2 portions.

1 portion contains 3 g protein, 0.6 g fat, 9.5 g carbohydrates, and 55 calories; with 2 tablespoons of coconut milk it yields a trace more of protein and carbohydrate, 1.8 g fat, 80 calories.

Peel the carrots, snip off the hard ends of the asparagus, wash the vegetables under running water, cut into small pieces, and cook for 5 minutes. Liquefy or puree the mixture in a blender. A small amount of coconut or almond milk may be added. When serving, garnish the soup with chopped green parsley or chives. You may also swirl (with a fork) a small amount of light sour cream in the center of the dish.

The soup can be stored in the freezer (without the sour cream).

Big Apple's Own (Waldorf) Salad

1/3 cup grapes
1/2 apple
1 stalk of celery
2 tablespoons walnut halves
1 tablespoon light mayonnaise
2 tablespoons fresh lemon juice
2 lettuce leaves

Makes one portion containing 2.3 g protein, 15 g fat, 57 g carbohydrates, and 373 calories.

Peel, core, and slice the apple, halve the grapes, and chop the celery and the walnuts. Mix the mayonnaise with lemon juice, and stir with the other ingredients. Place on lettuce leaves and top with walnuts.

Highly Vaunted Strudel

180 g flour
1 egg
100 g butter
4 tablespoons light cream cheese
3 tablespoons apple cider vinegar
1 teaspoon salt — not necessary if using salted butter
3 apples peeled, cored
3 tablespoons raisins
3 tablespoons slivered almonds or other chopped nuts
1 tablespoon cinnamon
1 teaspoon lemon rind

Makes 12 slices

1 slice yields 2.7 g protein, 10.5 g fat, 17 g carbohydrates, and 170 calories.

Preheat the oven to 170C (340F). Cut butter into small pieces (grate coconut butter or "shave" with a knife). Mix the first six ingredients, and knead briefly; some pieces of butter may show through the dough. Cut the pastry in two halves, and roll out each half into a 26 x 36cm (11" x 14") rectangle 2mm (1/8") thick. Roll it on a rolling pin, transfer to baking sheet, and unroll. Place the apple slices in the middle, sprinkle with cinnamon and grated lemon rind, top with almonds and raisins. Bring the two long sides of the pastry to the center so they overlap slightly. Pierce with fork. Repeat the process with the other half of the pastry. The baking sheet of the above mentioned size will accommodate two strudels. Bake until golden brown.

The strudel is naturally sweet, but may be dusted with icing sugar mixed with vanilla sugar just before serving. Strudel keeps well in freezer.

Alternate fillings may be used, such as prune or nut mixtures.

Prune filling:

20 large pitted prunes
1 tablespoon cinnamon
1 teaspoon grated lemon rind

Cut the prunes into small pieces, place in the middle of strudel, sprinkle with cinnamon and lemon rind.

1 slice of strudel with prune filling yields 2.7 g protein, 7.8 g fat, 20 g carbohydrates, and 160 calories.

Nut filling:

2 teaspoons flour
1/3 cup milk
200 g nuts, coarsely chopped or ground
5 tablespoons honey, molasses, maple or agave syrup
1 teaspoon grated lemon rind
1 tablespoon cinnamon
couple drops of pure almond extract
1/2 teaspoon salt

Briefly cook flour in milk till thickened. Remove from burner and mix in all ingredients. Place in the middle of rolled out pastry proceeding as mentioned in apple strudel recipe, or spread evenly on 2/3 of the pastry and make a roll.

1 slice of strudel with nut filling yields 5.3 g protein, 17 g fat, 22.5 g carbohydrates, and 265 calories.

Strudel with spinach filling is a tasty savory treat.

Spinach filling:

6 teaspoons butter
6 teaspoons flour
¾ cup milk
3 cups cooked spinach (from 6 cups fresh)
90g (3 ounces) 18% Swiss cheese

Use the basic strudel pastry recipe. Prepare the savory base recipe (found under crepes fillings) and mix in the cooked spinach and cheese. Roll out the strudel pastry, place the spinach mixture in the middle, and proceed as in the apple strudel recipe.

Makes 12 portions.

1 portion yields 5.8 g protein, 12.8 g fat, 15 g carbohydrates, and 198 calories.

Quick Comfort Bread Pudding

2 apples
2 teaspoons cinnamon,
1 teaspoon grated lemon rind
2 slices bread (raisin bread, multigrain bread or halved bagel)
1 tablespoon melted coconut or unsalted butter
2 tablespoons honey, maple or agave syrup

Makes two portions.

1 portion yields 2.7 g protein, 8.7 g fat, 41 g carbohydrates, and 250 calories.

Stew peeled, cored, sliced apples with cinnamon and pieces of lemon peel until tender. Remove the lemon peel. Toast the bread, spread with honey and melted coconut butter on both sides. Cut into smaller pieces, place half on the bottom of a serving dish, cover with stewed apple mixture, and top with the remaining bread. Serve hot or cold.

Mini Effort Crumble

100 g ground almonds
5 tablespoons honey
4 drops almond extract
1/4 cup chopped nuts (pecans, almonds, macadamia, pine, walnuts, cashews)
1/4 cup unsweetened fine coconut
4 tablespoons melted coconut or unsalted butter
dash of salt

Makes 6 toppings.

1 portion yields 4.5 g protein, 20 g fat, 19 g carbohydrates, and 275 calories.

Mix all the ingredients into a crumble (which can be stored in the freezer) and sprinkle on top of stewed or fresh fruit (apples, nectarines, peaches, pears, berries) just before serving. For a decadent touch, top with a little whipped cream or ice cream.

Going, Going, Gone Muffins

1/2 cup large oats
1 cup flour (durham wheat semolina, rye, spelt, or quinoa)
2 tablespoons baking powder
1 egg
1/2 teaspoon salt
1 teaspoon cinnamon
dash of ground cloves
1 teaspoon grated lemon rind
2 tablespoons chopped nuts
2 tablespoons raisins or chopped dried prunes
1 grated medium carrot
5 tablespoons honey/agave syrup
1 tablespoon molasses
4 tablespoons plain yogurt or buttermilk
3 tablespoons melted coconut oil

Makes approximately 12 muffins.

1 muffin yields 1.8 g protein, 6.2 g fat, 15.5 g carbohydrates, and 125 calories.

Grease the muffin cups, sprinkle oats on the bottom, or use paper baking cups. Mix all the dry ingredients together, then add the other ingredients, and mix well with fork or spoon. Fill 3/4 of muffin cups with the batter, and bake at 165C (330F) for approximately 25 minutes, or until a toothpick inserted in the middle of the muffin comes out dry. The muffins keep well frozen.

Invigorating Granola

2 cups of large rolled oats
1/3 cup oat bran
1/3 cup shredded unsweetened coconut
1/4 cup natural almonds with skin, chopped
1/4 cup pecans, chopped
1/4 cup walnuts, chopped
1/4 cup honey, agave or maple syrup
1/4 cup coconut oil
1/2 cup dried fruit of your choice (raisins, cranberries, apricots, pineapple, papaya, mango)
1/2 teaspoon of salt

1 heaping tablespoon of granola yields 1.1 g protein, 4.7 g fat, 9.8 g carbohydrates, and 88 calories.

Line the baking sheet with parchment paper and preheat the oven to 165C (330F). Heat the coconut butter and honey, mix well with all the ingredients (except for the dried fruit) and spread on top of the parchment paper. Occasionally stirring, bake for about 25 minutes or till the mixture is crisp. Let cool and stir in the dried fruit. Store in an airtight container.

Pest's Delight Truffles

5 tablespoons ground flax seed
5 tablespoons ground sesame seeds
5 tablespoons crunchy peanut or almond butter
2 tablespoons finely chopped juicy prunes
2 tablespoons finely or coarsely shredded unsweetened coconut
50 g bittersweet chocolate (72% cocoa)
1/4 cup finely chopped or ground nuts for coating

Makes 15 truffles

1 truffle yields 2.3 g protein, 7 g fat, 6.2 g carbohydrates, and 98 calories.

Melt chocolate on low heat and mix with all ingredients. Form into small balls, roll in nuts or unsweetened shredded coconut, and place in mini baking cups. Store in the freezer.

The number of servings as well as the nutrient and calorie count of each recipe are approximate.

Measurements and conversions

The values of the dry measurements in the following tables are approximate because the density of the ingredients varies. For instance, one cup of wheatlets weighs more than one cup of quinoa flakes; by the same token, three teaspoons of molasses may not always equal one tablespoon of milk.

Volume dry measurements:

1/4 teaspoon = 1.25 ml
1/2 teaspoon = 2.5ml
1 teaspoon = 5ml
1 tablespoon = 3 teaspoons = 15ml
1/4 cup = 4 tablespoons = 60ml
1/3 cup = 5 tablespoons = 75ml
1/2 cup = 7.5 tablespoons = 115ml
1 cup = 15 tablespoons = 230ml

Volume liquid measurements:

1 teaspoon = 5ml = 1/6 fluid ounce
1 tablespoon = 15ml = 1/2 fluid ounce
2 tablespoons = 30ml = 1 fluid ounce
1/4 cup = 60ml = 2 fluid ounces
1/3 cup = 79ml = 2 and 2/3 fluid ounces
1/2 cup = 118ml = 4 liquid ounces

1 cup = 250ml = 8 fluid ounces
2 cups (1/2 pint) = 500ml = 1/2 liter = 16 fluid ounces
4 cups (1 quart) = 1,000ml = 1 liter = 32 fluid ounces

Weight measurements:

1 ounce = 28.5 grams
4 ounces = 114 grams
8 ounces = 227 grams = 1/2 pound
16 ounces = 454 grams = 1 pound

Linear measurements:

1/2 inch = 1.25cm
1 inch = 2.5cm
4 inches = 10cm
10 inches = 25cm
20 inches = 50cm = 1/2 meter

Oven temperatures:

100 degrees Fahrenheit (°F) = 38 degrees Celsius(°C)
200 °F = 95 °C
250 °F = 120 °C
300 °F = 150 °C
350 °F = 180 °C
400 °F = 205 °C
450 °F = 230 °C

To convert Fahrenheit to Celsius:
subtract 32 from °F, multiply by 5, divide by 9.

To convert Celsius to Fahrenheit:
multiply °C by 9, divide by 5, add 32.

Suggested reading

A New Earth, Awakening To Your Life's Purpose, Tolle

Calm Focus Joy: The Power Of Breath Awareness, Thompson

Complete Food And Nutrition Guide, Duyff

Exercise And Physical Activity, National Institutes Of Health

Let Them Eat Vegan!, Burton

Nutrition For Canadians, Rinzler and Cook

Relaxation Revolution, Benson, Proctor

Sitting Kills, Moving Heals, Vernikos

Staying Healthy With Nutrition, Haas and Levin

The New Raw Energy, Kenton

True Food, Weil

Vegetarian, Heart

Yoga — The Path To Holistic Health, Iyengar

Yoga As Medicine, McCall